THE DANGER WITHIN US

THE DANGER WITHIN US

America's Untested, Unregulated Medical Device
Industry and One Man's Battle to Survive It

JEANNE LENZER

Little, Brown and Company
New York Boston London

Little, Brown and Company
Hachette Book Group
1290 Avenue of the Americas, New York, NY 10104
littlebrown.com

First Edition: December 2017

Little, Brown and Company is a division of Hachette Book Group, Inc. The Little, Brown name and logo are trademarks of Hachette Book Group, Inc.

The publisher is not responsible for websites (or their content) that are not owned by the publisher.

The Hachette Speakers Bureau provides a wide range of authors for speaking events. To find out more, go to hachettespeakersbureau.com or call (866) 376-6591.

ISBN 978-0-316-34376-3
Library of Congress Control Number: 2017954610

10 9 8 7 6 5 4 3 2 1

LSC-H

Printed in the United States of America

3 0646 00220 1089

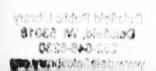

Contents

THE DANGER WITHIN US

Prologue

WHEN I WAS STUDYING to be a physician associate (PA) at Duke University, I was taught to diagnose and treat common and not-so-common illnesses. As a practicing PA, I wrote prescriptions, performed minor surgical procedures, and made referrals to specialists. I thought that if I stayed on top of new developments in medicine, and was caring and conscientious enough, I could help people. I wouldn't harm patients. Certainly I wouldn't kill them.

I was wrong.

For years, I worked in rural emergency rooms, serving as the sole on-site medical provider for patients with everything from sprained ankles to heart attacks and major trauma.

When I saw patients with chest pain, I routinely ordered several drugs, including one called lidocaine, given to prevent or stop extra heartbeats known as premature ventricular contractions (PVCs). Although PVCs can occur occasionally in healthy individuals and aren't dangerous in themselves, they tend to occur more frequently in heart attack patients, and they have the potential to touch off deadly heart rhythms.

Lidocaine was widely seen as a lifesaving drug. Professional organizations such as the American College of Emergency Physicians and the American Heart Association (AHA) had issued guidelines recommending lidocaine for routine use in patients with acute chest pain.[1] And like doctors across the nation, I had faith in the drug, not just because it was recommended but because I'd seen it save the life of a man too young to die.

Mr. R. was in his early forties when he was wheeled into the small rural ER where I was working as the medical provider along with two nurses. One of the nurses recognized him as a local firefighter. He had crushing chest pain and was sweating profusely. I saw the look of terror in his eyes and knew he was wondering, *Am I going to die?* Within minutes I had ordered oxygen, aspirin, nitroglycerin, and morphine for Mr. R. and was just about to add lidocaine when the alarm on his heart monitor suddenly emitted its high-pitched squeal. I looked up to see the fluorescent green tracing revealing a run of PVCs. I ordered the lidocaine, which the nurse injected into an intravenous line.

The first few minutes after a heart attack are always tense. If one of those PVCs touched off the deadly rhythm known as ventricular fibrillation, Mr. R. was likely to be dead within minutes. The nurse completed the injection. The PVCs persisted. As the alarm continued to screech, I felt beads of sweat collect on my upper lip. Finally the lidocaine took hold. The electrical storm was over. Mr. R.'s heart was beating normally. The alarm fell silent, and I exhaled.

The ability of lidocaine to magically erase these abnormal beats made me secure in the belief that I'd helped a patient cheat death. Over the years, I repeated this process for patients with chest pain many times. It felt good to save lives.

Until I found out I wasn't saving lives at all.

In the early 1990s, more than a decade after the AHA had

recommended lidocaine for chest-pain patients, studies with disturbing results began to emerge. In 1993, one author wrote in the *Journal of Emergency Medicine* that although the drug could reduce PVCs, "overall mortality may be increased."[2] A study sponsored by the National Institutes of Health called the Cardiac Arrhythmia Suppression Trial (CAST) found that, although oral drugs related to lidocaine, such as flecainide and propafenone, could suppress PVCs, if they *did* occur despite the medication, the PVCs were more likely to trigger deadly rhythms.[3] Researchers found that the patients who'd been medicated were actually 3.6 times more likely to die.[3] Thus lidocaine and related drugs could fix the PVCs but kill more patients than they saved in the process. To put it in the vernacular: the operation was a success, but the patient died.

When I learned about the lidocaine study, I was devastated. I was also fascinated. Could it be true that we were killing patients when we were eyewitnesses to so many cures? And if so, if we were really killing patients, why didn't we see the carnage we'd caused?

I began to search for answers. I stayed up late at night reading about clinical trials and statistics. I attended as many medical conferences as the dollars in my pocket allowed. The more I learned, the more obsessed I became. I wanted to know how and why it was possible for patients and doctors alike to become involved in this massive folie à deux, a dance in which everyone was convinced that the march of medical progress was saving lives even when it wasn't. How had the best and the brightest doctors, including the guideline writers at the American Heart Association, been fooled? And if we could be fooled by this class of drugs, how many other mirages were we chasing? How many more patients were we harming?

What I learned eventually led me to a very unusual doctor who was able to explain how and why medical illusions like the belief in lidocaine as a lifesaver arise: Dr. Jerome R. Hoffman, then a professor of medicine and emergency medicine at UCLA. Hoffman helped me understand how easy it is for healthcare professionals to make deadly errors despite their best intentions and advanced training, and I'll share a number of his insights later in this book. These revelations also led me to leave my career in medicine more than a decade ago to become an investigative medical journalist.

Since that time, and especially while writing this book, I've been stunned to learn how frequently complications produced by a medical treatment are mistaken for symptoms of the underlying condition—a phenomenon I refer to as *cure as cause*. The failure to consider a treatment or cure as the cause of a bad outcome means that when a patient dies following a heart attack, we assume that the death was due to the heart attack and not to the medicine we gave. Examples can be found in virtually every specialty, from emergency medicine to psychiatry, cancer care, infectious diseases, and more. Mistaking the ill effects of a treatment as symptoms of the condition being treated is an illusion that is both natural and understandable—and it's an illusion that the healthcare industry repeatedly exploits to reap enormous profits.

But I was in for yet another shock when I learned the untold story of medical devices and how they, too, can cause the very symptoms they are intended to cure. I began to delve into the rise of the medical device industry and its disturbing role in the healthcare business. Although many concerned citizens have grown distrustful of the pharmaceuticals industry, thanks to the high-profile exposés of dangerous drugs such as Vioxx and Avandia, the same skepticism is largely lacking about implantable devices—from simple devices such as the surgical mesh used for hernias and urinary incontinence to an array of more complex devices such as deep-brain stimulators; spine implants with biologically active bone stimulators; Wi-Fi-enabled pacemakers and defibrillators; breast implants; brain-fluid shunts; intrauterine devices; filters that catch blood clots on their way to the heart; lens implants for cataracts; cadaver bone used for dental surgery; artificial heart valves; gastric bands; artificial hips, knees, and elbows; hormonal implants; cochlear implants; radium seeds; stents to hold coronary, carotid, and renal arteries open; stents that release drugs; and more.[4-11] The public and doctors often perceive these devices as advanced products of cutting-edge technology that are inert and so, unlike drugs, don't have serious side effects.

Nothing could be further from the truth.

The reality is that the Food and Drug Administration (FDA) does not require manufacturers to submit even a single clinical trial for the overwhelming majority of high-risk implanted devices it approves.[12-14]* Whereas the standard for approval of a new medicine usually calls for two randomized controlled clinical trials, only *5 percent* of high-risk implanted cardiac devices have even partially met that standard.[13, 15] It's no wonder that many of the millions of patients who have been fitted with implanted medical devices have experienced little or no health benefit as a result—and that others have suffered serious, often fatal, complications from the implants themselves.

It wasn't long after I became known as a journalist that doctors and patients around the world began to contact me to share their experiences with unsafe drugs and dangerous devices. One story stood out—the story of a Texas man named Dennis Fegan who has spent years battling the after effects of a near-death experience linked to the supposedly safe medical device implanted in him by a well-intentioned doctor. I tell his story in this book not because it is the worst I've heard (it isn't) but rather because it reveals so much about what ails the medical device industry and, more broadly, the health-care system in the US.

As Fegan's story weaves throughout *The Danger Within Us*, powerful doctors at the epicenter of modern medicine appear, offering profoundly conflicting views that go to the heart of the way health-care is organized and our perception of what is science and what is

---

*   For more about this, see Chapter Three.

illusion in medicine. One of these doctors, Eugene Braunwald, the father of modern cardiology and emeritus professor of medicine at Harvard, has made discoveries that affect millions of people around the world.[16, 17] His career is emblematic of the changing face of healthcare and the emergence of what many call the medical-industrial complex, a network of wealthy and powerful institutions that has dramatically reshaped American healthcare over the past half century. Others, including Dr. Bernard Lown, a Nobel Peace Prize recipient and Harvard cardiologist,[18–22] and Hoffman, emeritus professor of medicine at UCLA,[23–28] have called for radical changes in our deeply flawed healthcare system. Their differing perspectives represent alternative future paths that policy makers, healthcare consumers, and concerned citizens urgently need to understand.

Many in the healing professions undoubtedly regret that their service to patients has become so enmeshed with the politics of healthcare and the ideological and partisan clashes it evokes. Yet from a broader perspective, such entanglement is all but inevitable. In the words of Rudolf Virchow, the brilliant nineteenth-century physician credited with bringing scientific rigor to medicine, "Medicine is a social science, and politics [is] nothing more than medicine on a grand scale."[29]

I hope the stories you'll read in this book will illustrate Virchow's insights, which suggest that we cannot achieve a healthy society solely through the application of medical and scientific knowledge and that we will need to address challenging questions about the organization of society, the distribution of resources, and access to information. The answers to these questions have profound implications about who we are as a people and what kind of society we want. Ultimately we have to decide whether healthcare should be treated as a commodity—or a common good.

Jeanne Lenzer
Kingston, New York
May 2017

Chapter One

STRANGE SEIZURES

DENNIS FEGAN WOKE UP with a start. He rolled over, pulling some covers with him as he scanned the darkness for his clock radio. Slowly his eyes focused on the tiny fluorescent lights telling him it was just a few minutes after 2:00 a.m. He flicked on a light, went to the laundry room, where he kept a calendar and a pen, and made a vertical mark under the date. It was July 2, 2006.

Fegan had trained himself to mark each seizure on his calendar to help his doctors manage his medicines. This night would prove unusually bad. He was awakened repeatedly by a pain in his throat. In a fog of fatigue and darkness, he eventually lost count of just how many seizures he had—but by morning there were a dozen marks on July 2, 2006.

Every Sunday for the previous fourteen years, Fegan, an imposing 48-year-old veteran of the hardscrabble Texas oil industry, had had brunch with his parents at the Town & Country Café in a small strip mall not far from Fegan's home, in Corpus Christi, Texas. This custom was his parents' way of keeping tabs on him ever since he'd

9

been diagnosed with epilepsy. But that morning when his parents called, Fegan told them to go along without him. He wasn't feeling well. Nothing serious. He just needed to get some sleep. He didn't mention that he was having a bad run of seizures.

As they finished brunch at the Town & Country Café, his parents, seated in a booth and served by their favorite waitress, Colleen, decided to bring some food to their son. They ordered the breakfast Fegan loved—egg-and-potato taquitos—to go, then drove over to the working-class section of town where he lived.

Fegan's parents, George and Irene, had been born and raised in Texas. Like most of their neighbors, they were "good Republicans," no-nonsense people who raised their children in a strict Catholic household. George was a geologist with the sprawling Texas oil industry. He was proud of his work and grateful for the stable income it provided. He and Irene liked both Presidents Bush, and they didn't hold much truck with people who were always harping about excessive corporate profits and the need for social welfare. Fegan had followed in his parents' footsteps. The last president he liked or paid any attention to at all was Ronald Reagan.

Irene knocked on the front door of Fegan's small, neat ranch house. When she got no response, George banged on the door. Finally they dug up a spare key they had and cautiously let themselves in. As they reached the small dining room, Fegan staggered out of his bedroom looking dazed. He peered at his parents, sat down at the dining-room table, and abruptly lost consciousness. Unable to reach him in time, George and Irene watched helplessly as Fegan fell sideways off his chair, slamming his head hard onto the uncarpeted floor.

Within a few minutes, Fegan roused, got up, and sat back down in the dining-room chair. Then, as if in a movie set to run in a sickening continuous loop, his parents watched the same scene all over again:

Fegan fell off the chair, this time slamming face-first onto the floor. Within a span of minutes, he awakened. Now fearful of another fall, he wiggled across the floor and propped himself up in a sitting position with his back against a wall and his legs splayed in front of him. His jeans were wet with urine. He looked half dead. And then he fell over again.

Fegan's cycles of passing out, waking up, and passing out again repeated like clockwork. His parents frantically dialed Fegan's neurologist, Dr. Juan Bahamon. Even though it was a Sunday morning, the doctor answered promptly and told them to dial 911 for an ambulance. He'd meet the family at the hospital. While they were waiting for the ambulance, Fegan told his parents he'd been having seizures since two that morning. Now, some ten hours later, Fegan's parents privately wondered how long he could last. They later learned their fears were not unwarranted.

By the time the ambulance arrived at Fegan's home, Irene and George Fegan had watched their son lose and regain consciousness at least eight times. The lead paramedic, believing Fegan was having seizures, injected diazepam, a drug commonly used to stop the life-threatening continuous seizures known as status epilepticus, directly into an intravenous line they'd placed in Fegan's arm. Surprisingly, the diazepam had no effect at all. Fegan continued to pass out and rouse at regular intervals. By then an ugly series of bruises was forming on Fegan's forehead from his falls. But the crew was too distracted by something else to pay attention to the bruises: when they hooked him up to a heart monitor, what they saw stopped them dead in their tracks.

Although he didn't yet know it, Dennis Fegan was already fatefully entangled in a complicated web of human error, corporate manipulation, and regulatory failure that would turn his life into a Kafkaesque nightmare—and that would encapsulate much of what is worst about the American way of healthcare.

★ ★ ★

The troubles of the US healthcare system are widely recognized. They have been the subject of countless articles, books, and television news stories. Politicians have debated their causes and possible cures for decades. Yet the seriousness of those problems, and the enormous price we pay in wealth, resources, and lives, are still not fully understood by most Americans. Consider a few of the appalling facts.

According to the Institute of Medicine (IOM), Americans today not only live shorter lives, they're also sicker than the people of virtually all other well-off nations.[30] And according to the United Nations, the US ranks number 43 in life expectancy, below Costa Rica and Cuba and just ahead of Lebanon.[31, 32] Life span has declined over the past two decades in the US for the first time since World War II.[33] Now, in 43 percent of US counties, women are no longer living as long as their mothers.[34–36]

Personal habits such as smoking and drinking are part of the cause of our shorter, sicker lives, but only a small part: Americans smoke and drink less than people in a number of peer countries.[37, 38] What the US *does* have compared to other wealthy nations are higher rates of violence, obesity, and drug use.[30] Only three nations included in the IOM report have higher homicide rates than the US: Mexico, Turkey, and Estonia.[30] But even these issues account for only a fraction of the excessive mortality in the US.

One huge problem is our squandering of resources on ill-advised treatments. The US spends trillions of dollars on healthcare each year, and 20 to 30 percent of that care is considered unnecessary.[39–41] Many treatments do significant harm beyond wasting resources: medical interventions (including implantation of medical devices) are now the third leading cause of death in the US, killing an estimated 225,000 to 440,000 Americans each year.[42] That's more deaths than from diabetes, murder, car accidents, and AIDS *combined*. By

2012, prescribed medicines, such as blood thinners and drugs for diabetes, were causing so many deaths that the nonprofit group Institute for Safe Medication Practices conducted a study to quantify the number of deaths and concluded that prescribed medicines are "one of the most significant perils to human health resulting from human activity."[43] Although the precise number of deaths from medical error, drug and device complications, and overtreatment is subject to debate, even if the numbers were cut in half they would still comprise the third leading cause of death in the US.

We also have a problem unheard of in other wealthy nations: a large uninsured and underinsured population, which is associated with an estimated 45,000 avoidable deaths per year.[44] Despite the promise of the Affordable Care Act of 2010 (often called Obamacare), unpayable medical bills continue to be the leading cause of bankruptcy in the US.[45-47] As we spend more and more each year on healthcare, we threaten not only patients' lives but also their personal finances and the nation's economy.

The causes of these devastating statistics are numerous and complex, with roots in politics, economics, and social and cultural forces. But at the heart of the problem is the growing wealth gap, which has a profound effect on life span, and a massive healthcare industry that is sapping our economy.[48-51] Healthcare is now the single biggest sector of the US economy. It is bigger than big oil, bigger than big banking, and bigger even than the famous military-industrial complex that President Dwight Eisenhower warned about in his farewell speech. In 2013, the most generous estimate pegged the price of the military-industrial complex at $1.3 trillion, while healthcare expenditures in 2015 were $3.2 trillion, consuming nearly one of every five dollars spent in the US.[52, 53]

We may be less healthy and long-lived than the people of dozens of other nations, but in one respect America comes first: we are number 1 in healthcare spending, far surpassing all other countries.

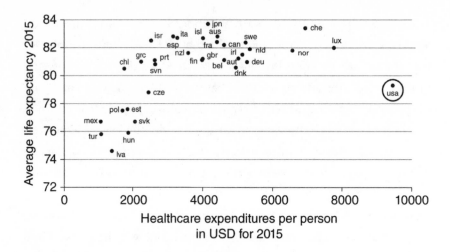

Life Expectancy vs. Healthcare Spending by Country, 2015.
Credit: Longevity from World Health Organization data; expenditures from the Organisation for Economic Co-operation and Development.

The poor performance of US healthcare strongly suggests that we are not getting what we should in exchange for this massive investment. And the wealth and power of the healthcare industry helps to explain why this is so. Over the past two generations—since the late 1960s—American healthcare has gradually been transformed from a relatively modest professional endeavor ruled mainly by traditional ethical norms governing independent doctors into a vast network of institutions dominated by for-profit corporations whose chief loyalty is to their shareholders and nonprofit organizations that function much as for-profit entities do.

While universities, government agencies, and some not-for-profit organizations such as certain hospitals and clinics continue to play an important role in developing, regulating, and administering healthcare treatments, they have been increasingly forced to follow the dictates of for-profit medical groups, hospital chains, insurance companies, drug manufacturers, and medical device makers, whose huge economic footprint translates into enormous political clout.

Taken together, this interlocking network of organizations makes up the medical-industrial complex. In October 1980, Arnold Relman, then editor of the *New England Journal of Medicine,* described "The New Medical-Industrial Complex," comparing it to the military-industrial complex, and said it posed "troubling implications."

The birth of the medical-industrial complex can be traced in part to the explosion of new healthcare technologies beginning in the 1950s and '60s, an era of healthcare innovation marked by the development of the first vaccines against polio, measles, and mumps.[54] The cardiopulmonary bypass machine first came into use in the early 1950s. Pacemakers, hip replacements, organ transplants, polymerase chain reaction, DNA fingerprinting, gel electrophoresis, stents for heart disease, and stem-cell therapy were all developed after 1960. CAT scans and MRIs were first performed on humans in 1971.[55] Commonly prescribed drugs exploded from a mere handful to many thousands, aimed at treating everything from high cholesterol to infections, restless leg syndrome, balding, overeating, and cancer.

Some of these innovations offer amazing benefits to the victims of age-old afflictions. Certain childhood forms of leukemia are now curable.[56] Infections that were previously life-threatening have been transformed into minor inconveniences. Diseased and worn-out human hearts, livers, and lungs can be replaced or tranplanted. The discovery of stem cells, the primordial cell type that gives rise to every other cell type—from hair to brain to liver and nerve—has brought researchers around the world close to developing lab-grown organs of every sort. Doctors have successfully implanted lab-grown skin, corneas, and bladders into human patients.

Some of the most recent breakthroughs have been so dazzling that they strain credulity. When an Internet image of a mouse growing a human ear on its back went viral, some viewers said it must have been digitally altered. It wasn't. The hairless laboratory mice running around in cages with ears on their backs were developed by Robert Langer, an MIT researcher, and Dr. Joseph Vacanti, director of the Laboratory for Tissue Engineering and Organ Fabrication at the Massachusetts General Hospital, in Boston.[57] The human-size ears, which take up almost the entire back of a mouse from neck to tail, begin life as a biodegradable ear-shaped scaffold, which the researchers seed with bits of cow cartilage. The structure is surgically implanted under the skin of "nude mice." The ears can be made to order for shape and size to match the needs of the human recipient.

The growth of complex body parts took a giant step forward in early 2008, when Doris Taylor created the first beating lab-grown heart.[58] Like Vacanti, she created a scaffold by dissolving the cellular material of a rat heart, then placing a mix of heart stem cells on the matrix. With careful environmental controls, the cells not only began to beat, they also even grew their own blood supply. "It's gorgeous," Taylor said of her creation. "You can see the whole vascular tree, from arteries to the tiny veins that supply blood to every single heart cell." By coupling lab-grown hearts with pacemakers, she hopes to create a supply of made-to-order, rejection-free human heart implants—a salvation for thousands of people who die each year while awaiting traditional transplants.

Can technology conquer death itself? It might seem reasonable to wonder these days. Researchers are studying telomeres, the little end plates on chromosomes that have been compared to the plastic tips on shoelaces that keep them from fraying. If the telomeres could be protected, chromosomes would never wear down and could duplicate forever, allowing humans to become immortal. The president of the American Academy of Anti-Aging Medicine, which on its website calls itself "the world's largest non-profit scientific society of physicians and scientists dedicated to the advancement of technology to detect, prevent, and treat aging related diseases," claims humans are "on the cusp of immortality."[59] Ray Kurzweil, described by the *Wall Street Journal* as "the closest thing to a Thomas Edison of our time," declares humans will be immortal by 2035.[60]

As these amazing examples illustrate, some medical break-throughs of the last sixty years have been impressive, even awe-inspiring, and genuinely important. They represent some of the finest achievements of an enormously wealthy and understandably self-confident American society at the height of its power and influence. But they also carry the seeds of serious trouble.

Today, like big oil and big banking, the medical-industrial complex has become so vast, so wealthy, and so powerful that it is increasingly insulated from the effects of its own errors and misdeeds. Virtually every major drug and medical device company has been caught in one or more scandals, and they pay massive fines as part of the cost of doing business.[61]

We often pay little attention to the companies that manufacture supposedly lifesaving drugs and medical devices until something goes wrong and we are suddenly caught up in the gears of the healthcare system. By then we may be too sick and scared to ask many questions. But whether we're paying attention or not, the inner workings of the medical industry touch our lives—literally. It's surprisingly easy for the products of profit-hungry companies to find their way into our bodies, whether they've proved safe and effective or not.

How did this happen? What is its impact on the lives of ordinary Americans? And what can we do about it? We can begin to understand some of the answers by returning to the story of Dennis Fegan.

Chapter Two

AGE OF MIRACLES

FROM HIS CHILDHOOD, DENNIS Fegan's family remembers him as a bit of a cutup. His sister, Catherine, says he was "funny and happy-go-lucky," with an adventurous, even mischievous nature that led to some early pranks. His mother, Irene, recalls that at just five years old, Fegan managed to get out of their fenced-in yard by pushing his tricycle up to the gate and standing on his tiptoes on the seat to open the latch (she figured this out only after she accused the water-meter reader of leaving the gate unlatched, but she was embarrassed and apologetic when she later saw her son attempting the stunt again). Once outside the gate, Fegan rode to a nearby supermarket, where he parked his tricycle in a parking space as if it were a car. Then he walked into the store, according to the manager, "just like he owned the place."

His pranks persisted long into his adulthood and would become the stuff of family lore.

In early May of 1965, Irene packed up the five Fegan children, ages two to eleven, in the family's 1954 Pontiac and headed to the

St. Patrick Catholic School to drop the older children off. As she entered an intersection, going through a green traffic light, she saw another driver entering from her left. She could see he was going to run a red light. "I knew I was going to be hit," Irene recalls. "I was standing on the brakes." But it was too late: the driver broadsided the left-side passenger area of the car, where her children were seated, sending the car into a spin.

The Fegan family's 1954 Pontiac had no seat belts. (It wasn't until 1959 that the first auto manufacturer installed them as standard equipment in their cars.) Dennis, then seven years old, was ejected from the backseat through an open window onto the street. When his family got to him, he was bleeding from his head.

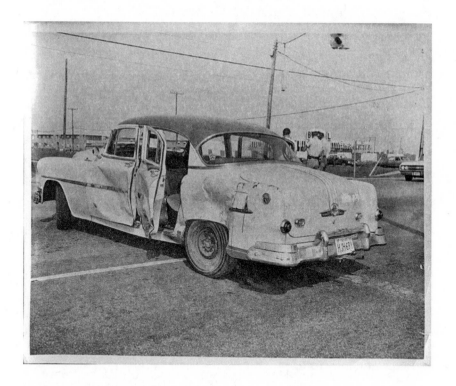

1965 car wreck that ejected Dennis Fegan, then 7 years old, through an open window, causing his head injury. (Photograph courtesy of the Fegan family)

Fegan has no memory of the accident itself, though he does remember waking up at Corpus Christi's Spohn Hospital, where doctors examined him. His medical record reveals that the doctors took
X-rays of his skull, knee, and shoulders. They noted a "deep laceration
with multiple hematomas" (bruises) over the right side of his head
and another half-inch laceration on his forehead. They sewed up the
lacerations with 4-0 silk, gave him a tetanus shot, and kept him in the
hospital for two days of observation. He did fine after his discharge,
and nothing further was made of the event for many years.

A strange incident occurred not long after the car accident. Neighbors of the Fegans were surprised to hear their doorbell ring late one
night. When they opened the door, they found seven-year-old Dennis
politely standing on their doorstep. He was stark naked. He had apparently sleepwalked to the house, where he stood waiting for someone
to come to the door. The neighbors were understanding and returned
the boy home. Fegan, forever humiliated by the incident, would sleep
in pajamas for the rest of his life, lest he ever sleepwalk again.

At age eleven, in 1969, Fegan watched in awe as Neil Armstrong
stepped onto the moon. He decided he would become an astronaut
and learn everything he could about NASA. But he had a backup
plan in case he couldn't make it as an astronaut: he'd become a
rock-and-roll star. Which required, of course, rebelling against his
parents' strict code of behavior. "I did everything I could to piss them
off," he says. "I wanted to be on my own, and I didn't want to follow
rules." And break the rules he did. As a teenager he started hanging
out with fast crowds, drinking beer and smoking pot, which caused
a fair amount of parental angst.

By the age of nineteen he was married, with a newborn child and
new expenses. His marriage didn't last, and he was separated from
his wife six years later. He says, "I was angry with Kathy for years
following the divorce because I laid all the blame on her. Actually, we
probably were both equally at fault. We were very young when the

children came along. Neither of us was mature enough to be starting a family." Kathy and Fegan remain on good terms, and he is close with his two sons, Michael and Derrick.

With children to support, Fegan decided to leave the small printing company where he worked after graduating from high school for a lucrative job as a roughneck in the hardscrabble world of the Texas oil industry. Soon he was scaling impossibly tall derricks. For the first week or so, the higher he climbed, the more afraid he became. But eventually, like other roughnecks who didn't give up or get killed, he became numb to the dangers and began scuttling about on the high platform as if he were on the ground.

Day in and day out, Fegan hauled heavy thirty-foot lengths of two-and-a-half-inch-diameter metal pipes to the top of the derrick and dropped them into the oil-well hole. Once at the top, he would tether his harness to safety ropes and lean out over an opening between the platform and the oil hole to drop the pipe in. This meant that for a few seconds he was essentially hanging, weighted by his cargo, over a straight drop from the top of the derrick to the concrete work floor some eighty feet below. A fall would mean certain death. It was hard and dangerous work, made all the more exhausting by the mind-numbing and incessant roar of the machinery.

One afternoon Fegan made his usual ascent and leaned forward to drop his pipe. Not unusually, he was standing at a do-or-die angle. The slightest extra tilt forward, or the slightest wind behind his back, would make it impossible for him to right himself, and if he lost his balance he would fall into the well hole just inches from his feet. Realizing the precariousness of his position, he reflexively put his hand behind him, reaching for the harness hook at the small of his back to assure himself that he was attached to a safety rope. His grasping fingers found the hook—but no rope. The blood drained from his head as he realized that when he'd returned from lunch, he'd forgotten to reattach his safety rope.

Studies by the Bureau of Labor Statistics report that the death rate for drilling workers is eight times the national average for all workers.[62] Roughnecks, who often work twelve-hour days, have the riskiest jobs on oil rigs. Fegan didn't know the statistics. He just knew that guys died on the rigs. In that terrible microsecond when he realized he wasn't tethered, he managed to jerk his upper body backwards, pulling himself upright onto the platform. His narrow escape left him shaking. But there was no time to fret over what happened; he had to keep the pipe moving. He kept working and comforted himself with the same thought that keeps many roughnecks going: there is always cold beer at the end of the day, when workers gather to unwind, drink away their jitters, and tell their stories with studied nonchalance, transforming their fear into boasts.

Dennis was changing from youthful rebel to responsible adult, yet the cheerful mischief maker remained. His brother Matthew recalls family get-togethers at their parents' house, where Fegan, his three brothers, and a gaggle of nieces and nephews would spend long Saturdays hanging out in the backyard:

> Thanks to Dennis, those days would eventually involve some kind of prank played on someone, usually Richard or George [Fegan's other two brothers]. My brother George liked to think of himself as a real macho tough guy, but if he wasn't careful he might end up driving back to Austin with some highly embarrassing bumper stickers affixed to his car. One time he drove away without realizing Dennis put two stickers on his rear bumper. One was a picture of Hillary Clinton. The other was a picture of [exercise celebrity] Richard Simmons, wearing his trademark tights. I remember George saying that if the mailman walked up to his house with some new magazine subscription that he had certainly not signed up for, he knew right away it was Dennis to blame.

Fegan made friends easily. Henry Gonzalez, a supervisor with the Corpus Christi Regional Transportation Authority, has been a close friend of Fegan's since tenth grade. They attended Mary Carroll High School in Corpus Christi together. Later they worked four different jobs together. After work they played cards and chess. Fegan, says Gonzalez, is a "super nice guy" who looked out for his friends and found them jobs when they needed work.

Christine Cobb Roderiquez, a friend of thirty-five years, knew Fegan through her uncle. She says, "Dennis stepped in when I lost my father...he has always been a very kind person. He loved to help people."

Work on the oil rigs took a toll, however. Although it paid well, it was exhausting, dangerous work, and it kept him away from his family. Within a few years, and with a second child on the way, Fegan decided to take a job closer to home. He went to school to become a paramedic and found a job with the Corpus Christi fire department. Eventually he rose to the position of captain.

In Corpus Christi, as in many other cities, emergency medical services are provided by the fire department. But in Corpus Christi, unlike some cities, paramedics are cross-trained as firefighters, and they alternate shifts, working one day as firefighters and the next day as paramedics. After Fegan was fully qualified as a paramedic, he underwent firefighter training, which involved an additional three months of intensive physical drills and book learning. He loved both jobs.

As a paramedic, Fegan was trained to administer a full line of emergency medicines, and the ambulance he worked in was also equipped with a state-of-the-art cardiac monitor that could transmit a patient's heart tracing (or cardiogram) in real time from the ambulance to doctors at the hospital who could guide the care of patients. If communications were lost, or for some reason a doctor wasn't immediately available, Fegan was trained to make decisions on his own, using approved protocols, in situations ranging from life-threatening asthma to out-of-control diabetes and instances of deadly status epilepticus, which Fegan had treated successfully on more than one occasion. He says, "Our goal was to get them there alive."

But a lot of emergency calls, says Fegan, weren't real emergencies. "We'd get calls from people who had a leg ache for a week and they think the ambulance is a taxi service." The problem was especially acute in the poor part of town, where many people didn't have a doctor or insurance, making the hospital emergency room their only source of healthcare.

Looking back many years later, he still vividly recalls one of the worst emergency calls:

We responded to a suicide report. We had a ride-along that day, a student paramedic. When we get to the scene, a man is lying [faceup] on the rug. He had an obvious gunshot wound in the middle of his forehead, and he had a .22-caliber gun in his hand. I didn't notice any breathing at first, and I told the student to go up to establish a level of consciousness. He gave the man a little shake, and the man sort of jumped and opened his eyes. Then I noticed that there was no exit wound and no pooling of blood. When we got him to the ER, the doctor said the forehead is the thickest part of the skull, and the bullet simply traveled around his head between the scalp and skull, and all he had to do was to make an incision and remove the bullet.

On another of the most disturbing calls, Fegan arrived at a house and found a young man hanging dead in a closet.

"The really gory, traumatic stuff," says Fegan, were the car accidents. He coped with the horror of these scenes the same way he coped with the dangers of being a roughneck: when it came to fear and trauma, he says, "I think I would just try to put that out of my mind. At the scene you have to concentrate on your job."

Some paramedics hesitated to go into certain parts of town, especially where shootings and assaults were more likely to occur, but Fegan says that while he was a little leery at first, he found "everyone treated me with respect. I never had a problem with anybody, even in the worst part of town."

Fegan may not have had a problem going into high-crime areas, but he had a close brush with death while fighting a fire once. He was decked out in full gear, wearing his helmet, full face mask, and the heavy suit known as a bunker suit, along with an air pack on his back. The oxygen supplied by an air pack is usually enough to allow a firefighter to breathe for thirty minutes. Fegan recalls,

We were inside this large house. The air pack gives you a warning if you're close to running out of oxygen. I got the warning, and I knew I had to get out of the house fast. But the house was so large, and I couldn't see because of all the smoke, so I kind of got lost. In these situations you're supposed to follow the water hose by straddling your feet on either side of the hose and feeling your way out. But the hose made some loops, and I didn't know if I was going to end up at the nozzle end of the hose or the front door. I knew I'd be dead if I didn't make the right choice. And just as I did get to the door, the air pack ran out.

You can get exhausted. A lot of people, after fighting the fire for a while and wearing all the heavy gear, have to get out of the building. You fight until you can't fight any more. And you're not criticized for it. But I never had a problem where I'd have to leave. After working in the oil fields, sometimes working up to twelve hours a day, I was in good shape.

Fegan's work was tough, but he enjoyed it. For him, fighting fires was a "fun challenge." His son Derrick remembers feeling proud of his father's job, saying, "When he brought his turnout gear home you could smell smoke on it. And that became a passion of mine. I thought: *I want to do that.*" (Derrick, who is now thirty-one, eventually did follow in his father's footsteps and became a paramedic and a volunteer firefighter in Austin, Texas.)

Around the time that Fegan became a captain in the department, Henry Gonzalez noticed a change coming over his friend. "I remember being with him at his house while he was studying to become captain," he says. "We were chatting, and all of a sudden his conversation took a turn and he wasn't making any sense...his words were clear, but he wasn't making complete sentences...it went on for about fifteen minutes, and then he started to make sense and then he'd say, 'Now, what was I talking about?'"

Then one morning, after pulling a twenty-four-hour shift at his paramedic job, Fegan got in his Isuzu pickup truck to drive home. He has no idea what happened, but somewhere along the way he blacked out. When he came to, he was parked at a haphazard angle outside a stranger's house, groggy and confused. He'd apparently made it most of the way home, and when he blacked out his truck had rolled to a stop on the slight upward incline of a neighbor's driveway. As he awakened, he says he realized his tongue was "bloody and nearly bitten off." He pulled himself together and drove home. Then he called his doctor.

Fegan's doctor listened to his story and concluded that he'd probably had a seizure. He wasn't sure just why, but he suggested it might be from too much drinking. Fegan reckoned he might be right. He did like his beer, and would sometimes drink eight to twelve cans a day. So he quit. Just stopped. Nonetheless, he had another seizure. That time he'd been dry for six months.

After the second seizure, his doctor prescribed phenytoin, a first-line drug for seizures, and told him he couldn't drive anymore. He was put on light duty at work. Soon he was having a new type of seizure—odd episodes where he'd "phase out." Once, his father noticed his arms jerking while he remained sitting up. His sister, Catherine, says he "just looked deep in thought" during his episodes. She recalls, "He'd seem to glance down. He wouldn't look you in the eye. Then it looked like he was chewing the inside of his cheek. Once, he put his hands up as if to say, 'Excuse me'—and then he was out of it."

Fegan's neurologist explained to him that he had temporal lobe epilepsy, which can cause "complex partial seizures"—a form of epilepsy that can cause odd symptoms.[63, 64] (Sometimes temporal lobe seizures can trigger grand mal seizures, and Fegan was plagued by both.) Partial seizures aren't like grand mal seizures, the sort most people associate with "epilepsy." Grand mal seizures cause people to lose consciousness, fall down, and shake violently as an electrical firestorm sweeps over most or all of the brain. A person in the grip of a grand mal seizure often loses control of his or her bowel or bladder.

The rogue electrical impulses of temporal lobe epilepsy, on the other hand, affect only a small portion of the brain, allowing other areas to continue to function—albeit in a potentially altered fashion. Vision, speech, and the ability to walk might be preserved during a temporal lobe fit. The manifestations of the seizures can vary widely, making temporal lobe epilepsy difficult to diagnose, because doctors generally have to rely on a patient's or witness's description of the episode. Individuals in the throes of a complex partial seizure might walk aimlessly from one room to another. They might make odd, repetitive, and useless gestures known as stereotyped movements (like chewing the inside of the cheek repeatedly, as Fegan's sister had observed him doing). They might look as if they are repeatedly and ineffectively reaching for something or attempting to straighten out an article of clothing. Sudden bursts of rage and psychotic episodes can also occur. But perhaps the most puzzling effect of a temporal lobe seizure is the strange fuguelike state of consciousness that some individuals experience, a state in which they appear suspended between full alertness and a dreamlike netherworld.

Whatever the cause, over time, it was hard to find the right combination of medicines to control Fegan's seizures, and he became one of the roughly 20 to 40 percent of people with epilepsy who are "treatment resistant"—individuals whose seizures are poorly controlled with medicine.[65, 66] So the calendar where Fegan kept a record of his seizures was especially important: his doctor consulted it and adjusted the types and doses of medicines he prescribed for him accordingly.

Even without changes in his drug regimen, the number of seizures Fegan had could vary wildly. One month he might have a dozen seizures a day, for many days. Another month, he'd go days or weeks with no seizures at all. It wasn't easy to manage his medicines. After a while there were so many pills that it could be hard to remember to take them all, and the side effects could make him feel groggy and slow, as if he were trying to move through quicksand.

The events following Fegan's early seizures unfolded with ferocious speed. His friend Gonzalez describes Fegan's transformation: "He went from having a good job, a job he loved, to no job, no car, no driver's license—and now he has to walk to the grocery store. He became very apprehensive to go anywhere. I think he was more afraid of someone seeing him have a seizure than he was of hurting himself." It wasn't long before Fegan's seizures started to take a toll on his personal relationships. Unable to drive and forced to retire from his career as a paramedic and firefighter, he began to withdraw, avoiding going out to see people.

Roderiquez, his friend of thirty-five years, also noticed the changes in Fegan's personality over time. Before the seizures, she says, "Almost every day we could we'd go to the beach, go jogging, hang out, drink beer.... We'd go to clubs and we'd dance; we loved to dance. We'd go out with my uncle's friends, and they always looked out for me, especially Dennis. He has a heart of gold." But, she says, after the seizures started, her friend retreated. They didn't go to the beach or out dancing. Fegan stayed inside and kept to himself.

Fegan's son Derrick recalls the day when his dad's seizures forced him to retire from the fire department. He had seen his father as a man who ran into burning buildings to save people, a man who would brave dangerous situations as a paramedic to save lives. Now he seemed afraid to leave the house. Derrick didn't understand what was happening to his father at the time, and his behavior made the younger man feel angry and confused.

Fegan didn't tell anyone about his fear of having a seizure in public—not even his family. When he failed to show up with his sons as promised for a family Christmas gathering, his parents and siblings were hurt, even offended. Like a tortoise slowly retracting its legs and head into its shell, Fegan was becoming a recluse—and his bewildered family didn't understand why.

His mother had a theory about his seizures. "I'd blame them on the beer, and I had no sympathy," she says. What else could explain his behavior? Matthew, too, thought his brother's problem was related to drinking. But after a few extended visits with Dennis, Matthew says he realized that his brother had a genuine medical problem: "I would come in for the weekend, and I'd be there all day long...and he's in [my] presence the whole day and [I] know he's had nothing to drink, but his behavior was so much like someone who was drunk or hungover."

It is not surprising that Fegan's complex partial seizures were misread. In the late 1800s, famed British neurologist John Hughlings Jackson described the mental state of individuals experiencing a temporal lobe seizure as a "dreamy state" in which he or she might have a "double consciousness" with vivid hallucinations, as if a dream were intruding on the waking, conscious state. Such individuals could seem drunk or crazy—or even appear to be simulating or faking a problem.[67] Many patients with complex partial epilepsy are referred to psychiatrists, because doctors as well as family members fail to recognize the condition as epilepsy.[67, 68]

On the less common occasions when Fegan would have a grand mal seizure, bystanders would immediately recognize the problem. But most of the time his seizures were so subtle that it would be difficult even for a careful observer, or Fegan himself, to know what was happening. He says, "I might be standing in a checkout line at a grocery store and the next thing I know, other people in the store are asking me if I'm okay." At these times, Fegan would go into the fuguelike state described by John Jackson. He wouldn't fall down. He wouldn't lose consciousness in the ordinary sense. And other than sometimes appearing to be chewing the inside of his cheek, he didn't shake or make any unusual movements that might signal a seizure. It was as if he were experiencing intermittent episodes of suspended animation.

Despite treatment with multiple medicines, Fegan's seizures persisted, and he began to look around for other options. His neurologist, Dr. Juan Bahamon, referred him to a doctor in another town, a two-hour drive from Corpus Christi, where he could be evaluated for possible brain surgery. If doctors can identify the area of the brain that is triggering seizures, known as the epileptogenic focus, surgically removing that small part of brain can be an effective treatment.

Fegan underwent a battery of tests, including a video electroencephalogram (video EEG), a test that combines a brain-wave test with video of a patient to detect seizure activity in relation to brain-wave changes. The tests told the story: six areas in the right temporal lobe of Fegan's brain were misfiring. And there was a possible focus deep in his brain stem, an area too dangerous to cut.

Since he wasn't a candidate for surgery, Fegan asked Bahamon for help. Wasn't there something else that could be done? Bahamon told him about a last-ditch option: the vagus nerve stimulator (VNS) device. No one was quite certain how or why shocking the vagus nerve could control seizures. But according to Cyberonics, the company that manufactured the device, the VNS was effective and safe, usually causing only minor side effects such as a cough or hoarse voice. Cyberonics had won FDA approval to market it as a treatment for epilepsy just three years earlier, in 1997.[69]

For Fegan, the decision was a simple one. He trusted his doctors and didn't second-guess their recommendations. Eight years after he was first diagnosed with epilepsy, in June of 2000, at the age of forty-two, he underwent implantation with the VNS device.

The neurosurgeon implanted the device by first making two incisions, one under Fegan's left collarbone and another at his neck, near his carotid artery. He then tucked the matchbox-sized device just below Fegan's collarbone and tunneled two wire leads from the device up to his neck, where he carefully wrapped the wires around Fegan's vagus nerve. During the operation, the neurosurgeon tested the device by triggering small electrical shocks to the nerve. It delivered the tiny shocks as expected.

To Fegan, the surgery was no big deal. He was, after all, a former oil-rig worker, a fighter of fires, a guy who had for years been at the mercy of debilitating seizures. The device, he figured, could only make life better. His incision sites healed up nicely, and the electrical component of the device was switched to Off for the first two weeks following surgery—a standard approach to allow the vagus nerve to recover from being manipulated and encircled with wires. When the device was turned on again, he didn't have any of the common side effects caused by the device. He didn't cough. His voice wasn't hoarse.

It appeared as if Dennis Fegan was simply the latest beneficiary of one of the miraculous technological cures that modern medical science was steadily producing to alleviate the suffering of countless victims of disease. Neither Fegan nor his healthcare providers had any idea that the implantation of the VNS device would prove to be the start of a disastrous downward spiral that would all but destroy his life.

* * *

It's likely that very few of the tens of thousands of patients who have vagus nerve stimulators in their bodies have ever wondered about the experimental origins of the device. Even most physicians who recommend and implant the device have little knowledge of the science behind it. But the story of the VNS device is a fascinating and revealing illustration of how, in the last three decades, scientific breakthroughs have been converted into technological tools and then, at an accelerated pace, into moneymaking products.

The story begins with Dr. Eugene Braunwald, arguably *the* golden boy of modern American medicine. His biographer and colleague, Harvard cardiologist Thomas H. Lee,[*] says Braunwald is more responsible than any single individual for the dramatic transformation of medicine that began in the second half of the twentieth century.[17] Lee writes, "Since the 1950s, the death rate from heart attacks has plunged from 35 percent to about 5 percent—and fatalistic attitudes toward this disease and many others have faded into history. Much of the improved survival and change in attitudes can be traced to the

---

[*]   Lee worked for Braunwald and, as such, may not be an objective observer.

work of Eugene Braunwald, M.D. By redirecting cardiology from passive, risk-averse observation to active intervention, he helped transform not just his own field but the culture of American medicine."[17]

Braunwald was an overachiever from a very early age, and it seemed preordained that he would rise to the top of any field he entered. Born in Vienna, Austria, on August 15, 1929, he described his childhood as "idyllic."[16, 17, 70, 71] His parents began taking him to the opera when he was just five—a pleasure he continued to enjoy throughout his life. "I felt totally secure," he said. "I had private piano lessons, I had an English tutor, and I went to a very good school...my mother would take me to the park and I would be in my Lord Fauntleroy outfit, including the white gloves. The University of Vienna was just two or three blocks away. We would take a walk, and she would point to the University and say, 'You're going to be a professor here.'"

In school he showed a fierce drive to succeed. While other youngsters his age took welcome breaks from school and homework, Braunwald shuttered himself in his room, studying with a single-mindedness that set him apart. Even family gatherings and games failed to lure him away from his studies.

Braunwald's family narrowly escaped the Nazis, moving first to London and then to New York in 1939, when he was a child. Four years after the family settled in Brooklyn, Braunwald had adapted to his new environment well and was an outstanding student. He graduated first in his eighth-grade class, and in 1944, at the age of fourteen, he won admission to Brooklyn Technical High School, an elite school focused on engineering, math, and science. He raced through his course work, ultimately opting for a "diploma mill" to graduate, then, at sixteen, he began college at New York University. By his own account he studied "about a hundred hours per week," earning straight As. It was at NYU that he would meet his future wife, Nina Starr, who would go on to become the first female heart surgeon. His sole escape from long hours of study was to sneak off to the opera with Nina.

Although he originally wanted to be an engineer, he realized he lacked the manual dexterity required to do drafting and shop work. So he switched his career goals and decided to go into medicine. Once again, Braunwald leaped ahead in his studies. At the age of nineteen, just two years after starting college, he entered NYU's medical school. In 1952, he received his MD, graduating first in his class. As an intern, he recalls, "I read when other people were too tired to read." He was on his way to becoming one of the most well-known men in medicine.

After considering a number of specialties, he ultimately settled on cardiology, a field he said was closest to engineering: "In cardiology, I deal with pumps, which is like mechanical engineering. But I also deal with electricity, so there's a bit of electrical engineering, too."

While excited by the challenges, Braunwald was also troubled by some of the practices he saw as a medical student. Early in his training, he recalls walking to Bellevue Hospital and seeing doctors in their white lab coats hurry past homeless people lying on the street. Later, while in training as a resident at Johns Hopkins Hospital, he had his first encounter with segregated wards. There were two separate training programs: doctors in training in the Marburg service provided care to private patients, while those in the Osler service provided care to all patients. Braunwald applied only to the Osler service. Patients were segregated there, too, in four large wards divided by race and sex. Even blood was segregated, and Braunwald was disturbed that although the blood of white donors could be given to African Americans, the reverse was not true. The concept of a white person's "racial purity" being "contaminated" by black blood was likely evocative of his narrow escape from the Nazis as a child.

Despite the blatant class and race divisions at Johns Hopkins, Braunwald was impressed that all patients were addressed as sir or Mr.

or Miss or Mrs.—but never by their first names, as was so often the case at other hospitals (unless the patient was a well-off white male).

Medical research was Braunwald's greatest passion. At the impossibly young age of twenty-eight, he became chief of the section of cardiology and subsequently the clinical director of the National Heart and Lung Institute, which in later years became part of the federally funded National Institutes of Health (NIH). His arrival there coincided with what are often called the golden years of the NIH: 1955–1968. Funding soared during that period, rising from about $100 million to more than $1 billion per year. The NIH was an exciting and prestigious perch, and Braunwald reveled in his research collaborations with other scientists there.

Yet in many ways, medical research was still in its infancy, with few doctors trained in research methods, and Braunwald wanted to bring some of his training at the NIH to the broader medical community. So in 1968 he left the NIH to become the first chairman of the department of medicine at the University of California San Diego School of Medicine, where he hoped to create what he called triple threat physicians—doctors who could teach, conduct research, and practice bedside medicine.

In another step up the ladder, he moved back to the East Coast in 1972 to become a professor of medicine at Harvard Medical School. That same year, he served on the President's Advisory Panel on Heart Disease. The living Nobel Prize winners in physiology or medicine named him the "person who has contributed the most to cardiology in recent years."[72] He wrote more than twelve hundred scholarly articles and served as the editor of the primary textbook used by medical students and doctors around the world: *Harrison's Principles of Internal Medicine.* He remains the editor of *Braunwald's Heart Disease,* which is widely considered the bible of cardiology.[16, 17, 70, 71]

One of the many young physicians whose lives were affected by Eugene Braunwald was Jerry Hoffman, who met Braunwald in 1970 at the UCSD School of Medicine. Hoffman recalls his first impression of Braunwald: "I had no doubt at all that he was brilliant and incredibly accomplished. In virtually every aspect of cardiology he had made enormous, seminal contributions. He was in some ways an excellent teacher as well as such a giant figure in American medicine. I've never forgotten the lessons he taught us about cardiac pathophysiology because he made the concepts—many of which were based on work he himself had done—clear and understandable."[*]

But Hoffman also recalls of Braunwald:

He was imperious, and certainly no one would have dreamed of talking back to him or questioning anything he said. His personal manner was extremely cold and off-putting, and he tolerated not even a hint of a challenge to authority—which I have long since come to believe is a terrible barrier to real learning. I'm pretty sure most if not all of us—residents and fellows and even faculty as well as bottom-of-the-pile students like me—felt not merely intimidated but actually demeaned by the way he talked down to us.

Hoffman never forgot the lecture Braunwald delivered on angina pectoris—the name for chest pain associated with coronary artery disease:

Angina was obviously a very important topic—and the lecture was given by Braunwald himself. So there we were seated in the auditorium, in our little white jackets, and everybody was nervous in front of Braunwald, who was always so stern. He brought in one of his patients, a retired navy admiral, to show us how to take a history from a patient with chest pain. There was

---

[*] From a phone interview with Hoffman on May 28, 2013.

one student in our class who always read ahead so that he could ask questions to show that he already knew more than was expected of us. He'd obviously read about how heart disease could interfere with physical activity—including sexual activity—so he asked the admiral something about his sex life. The admiral responded with a little joke, and everyone laughed. It was a nice moment and a relief from the general tension that was always considerable when Braunwald was at the podium.

But after the admiral left the room, Braunwald ripped us a new asshole. He told us how humiliating and puerile our behavior was, tittering like little children about sex—he let us know in no uncertain terms how ashamed of us he was.

During the lecture, Braunwald had made a point of teaching the students about the so-called Levine sign, a classic gesture made by patients who have coronary chest pain to describe their symptom. He asked the admiral to point with one finger to the place where his chest hurt. But instead the admiral balled up his fist and placed it over the center of his chest, saying it wasn't in just one spot. Braunwald exclaimed, "That's it—Levine's sign! When he put his hand to his chest like that and turned it into a fist, covering an entire area. If there's one thing I want you to remember from this lecture, it's what it means when a patient makes a Levine sign."

After the lecture, Hoffman and a friend found themselves waiting for an elevator with Braunwald and his cardiology fellow, who was furiously brownnosing Braunwald. Hoffman says, "He was telling Braunwald what a fabulous, wonderful lecture he had given and that none of us would ever, *ever* forget the Levine sign."

Hoffman waited a few beats, then turned to his friend and said in a stage whisper, "What was that thing, you know . . . that the patient did with his fist?"

Braunwald was not amused. "He turned around and glared at me, and it was clear that if he could have crushed me at that moment, like the cockroach he surely considered me to be, he would have."

Jerry Hoffman's irreverent bit of nose thumbing revealed an iconoclastic side to his own personality that we'll encounter again in a very different context later in this book. But the story also shows us something about Eugene Braunwald—a brilliant, innovative medical thinker not greatly endowed with the gifts of humor, humility, or self-doubt... which may help explain some of the unfortunate byways into which he would later wander and into which he would help steer a significant portion of the American medical establishment.

Braunwald did much more than simply conduct his own program of medical research. In 1984, he founded the Thrombolysis in Myocardial Infarction (TIMI) Study Group, which would grow into a multibillion-dollar multinational research organization with eight thousand researchers in fifty-two countries and more than three hundred thousand human test subjects enrolled in clinical trials.[73, 74] Braunwald seemed to be everywhere, and his accomplishments were praised as unparalleled.

His most important research contributions have been in four areas: diseases of heart valves, heart attack, an unusual condition now known as hypertrophic cardiomyopathy (HCM), and congestive heart failure.

The discovery of HCM resulted from one of the most frightening moments of Braunwald's career.[17] Back in 1958, he had been working on aortic valve disease at the National Institutes of Health, the epicenter of medical research in the US, with Andrew Glenn Morrow, a heart surgeon. The aortic valve keeps oxygenated blood flowing forward from the left side of the heart to the rest of the body. If the valve becomes hardened and stiff, it restricts the forward flow of blood, depriving the brain and body of oxygen. The result can be chest pain, congestive heart failure, syncope (passing out), and even death if it is left untreated.

Sometimes the aortic valve fails to close properly after the heart contracts, allowing blood to flow in the wrong direction, back into the heart, also depriving the brain and body of oxygenated blood. Less commonly, a fibrous ring just below the aortic valve can interfere with the forward flow of blood. Each of these malfunctions causes distinctive changes in the pressure gradients inside the heart. By measuring the pressures, Braunwald and Morrow could determine the diagnosis. Morrow depended on Braunwald's findings to plan the appropriate operation.

But all seemed to go horribly wrong one summer day in 1958, when Morrow angrily summoned Braunwald to the operating room. Braunwald arrived to find a young man lying on the operating table, his rib cage cut and his chest splayed open. His heart, an organ never meant to be exposed to the external world, was on display: red and still—paralyzed by a flood of potassium that was allowing Morrow to perform surgery. The man's blood was being pumped through a cardiopulmonary bypass machine that artificially oxygenated his blood.

As the young man lay unconscious on the operating table, Morrow said, "There's a terrible screw-up here. I opened this guy's heart, and I just can't find anything wrong with it."

Braunwald was confused. He recalled listening to the patient's loud heart murmur and hearing that he was short of breath prior to surgery. He had analyzed the pressure tracings from the patient's cardiac catheterization. The pressure gradient indicated some sort of obstruction just below the aortic valve.[16]

Yet when Morrow opened the man's chest, the aortic valve itself was normal—and when he poked his finger through the valve, to the subaortic area, there was no evidence of a fibrous ring. *Nothing was wrong.*

Braunwald was horrified. It was as if he had sent the wrong patient to surgery. Worse, in 1958, getting a patient's heart restarted was not a sure thing. These were still the early years of cardiopulmonary bypass, and the techniques of stopping and restarting the heart were in their infancy. The bypass machine, developed in the early 1950s, had such a poor record initially that William S. Stoney, a cardiothoracic surgeon, reported in the prestigious medical journal *Circulation*: "The first attempts at cardiopulmonary bypass during those years were a series of disasters with an appalling mortality rate. During [the] four years between 1951 and 1955...of the 18 patients reported to have had an operation using cardiopulmonary bypass at 6 different centers...[there was] only 1 survivor."[75]

To lose a patient during a necessary surgery was one thing; to lose a young man who never needed surgery in the first place would be devastating.

Braunwald felt sick.

As Braunwald left the operating theater, he made a plea: If Morrow could get the young man's heart beating again, would he please stick a needle in the man's left ventricle to see if Morrow observed the pressure gradient Braunwald had found during his catheterization?

Morrow did manage to get the man's heart restarted, and when he did, he fulfilled Braunwald's request. He pierced the left ventricle with the needle, and to his surprise, he found the abnormal pressure gradient Braunwald had reported earlier. But the finding was puzzling. There was no obstruction. How could this happen? The two men had no way to explain it.

Shortly after this incident, other patients began to present with the same mysterious problem. Morrow noticed something: although these patients didn't have any fixed obstruction that could be seen or felt, they did have an unusual thickening of the heart muscle just below the aortic valve. Instead of a fibrotic, or hard and calcified, lesion, what he found was a hypertrophied, or enlarged, muscle that would squeeze so effectively that it created a dynamic obstruction that could be observed *only as the heart was beating*.

In 1959, Morrow and Braunwald published their findings in *Circu-*

lation and named their discovery idiopathic hypertrophic subaortic stenosis, or IHSS.[76] Later they would discover that the condition had a genetic component, and the term *idiopathic*—meaning of unknown cause—was dropped. Ultimately the condition was renamed hypertrophic cardiomyopathy, or HCM. Their work led to new medical and surgical treatments for HCM, which is estimated to affect one in five hundred people.

Looking back many years later, Braunwald called his work on this condition "the most exciting of my professional life."[70]

Braunwald, now in his eighties, speaks in a gravelly voice with a thick Boston accent. His work on HCM may have been especially exciting, but his greatest achievement, he says, was his insight into the nature of heart attacks and his discovery that their severity could be modified. This was a novel concept at the time, and it came about from one of the most dramatic "aha" moments of his career—a moment that would change how doctors understand heart attacks and would ultimately lead to new treatments for the number one killer in the US... and to the VNS device that would be implanted in Dennis Fegan in 2000.

Braunwald's moment of insight came during a chance meeting after he gave a guest lecture in 1967 in Rochester, New York. He was preparing to leave to catch his plane home when Seymour Schwartz, the author of the leading textbook on surgery, approached him. Schwartz asked if he'd be interested in seeing his experiments in treating high blood pressure, which he conducted on dogs. Braunwald agreed and accompanied Schwartz to the dog lab.

In order to treat high blood pressure, Schwartz first had to create high blood pressure in the dogs, which he did by surgically removing one kidney from each dog. Then he wrapped the remaining kidney in cellophane, causing it to release renin, an enzyme that triggers a cascade of hormones that regulate blood pressure. Once the dogs became hypertensive, he rigged up a crude electrical device similar to a pacemaker that delivered small shocks to wire leads protruding from the dogs' necks. The wires were wrapped around the carotid sinus nerves, which are activated via stretch receptors in the carotid sinus, a small swelling in the carotid artery that senses blood pressure. The carotid sinus loop involves a feedback mechanism that stimulates the vagus nerve, slowing the heart rate, weakening the force of the heart's contractions, and dilating blood vessels. This triad of effects causes blood pressure to drop, thereby treating the dogs' artificially induced hypertension. If the device worked, said Schwartz, it might be possible to use it to treat high blood pressure in humans.

This gave Braunwald an idea: since the electrical stimulator effectively decreased blood pressure, it could theoretically reduce the workload of the heart. If that was the case, perhaps it could be used to treat not just high blood pressure but also heart pain, known as angina.

In an interview with the *Journal of Clinical Investigation* posted on YouTube, Braunwald relates how he and his wife, Nina, developed a carotid sinus or vagus nerve stimulator that patients could activate themselves if they had chest pain:[16]

I came home that evening, and I said to Nina, "Do you think that you could implant [a] carotid sinus nerve stimulator into patients?" And she said, "Why? What for? That sounds nutty to me." So I told her about the [visit with Schwartz], and she said, "Yeah, I think I could do it." And…she went to the autopsy room and learned how to dissect out the human carotid sinus nerves…and that isn't something that is that easy to find.

Research was so different at that time. From the conception of the idea at Rochester to the time the first patient was implanted was six weeks. Now it would probably take six years going through committees and through all sorts of hurdles. Anyway, it helped. It was an excellent way for patients to turn the stimulator on themselves.

In a gutsy experiment in 1967, Braunwald became the first doctor to implant humans with a medical device—a prototype of the VNS—to treat angina.

Within months of his visit to the Schwartz lab, Braunwald published an article in the *New England Journal of Medicine* describing the "striking relief" experienced by two men in their fifties, an artist and a drug salesman, after he implanted them with a stimulator device. The very next year, in 1968, one of his patients with a stimulator came to the clinical center at the National Institutes of Health with severe chest pain. Worried that the man was in the throes of an impending heart attack, Braunwald cautioned him not to activate his stimulator. He worried that turning the device on during an actual heart attack—as opposed to when he was experiencing uncomplicated chest pain—could increase the likelihood of dangerous heart rhythms. To Braunwald's chagrin, despite "evidence of an ongoing heart attack," his patient "didn't listen" to his advice. He recalls:

> When I came to see him in the coronary care unit I found he had it on, and I turned it off. I came back to see him about every twenty minutes, and several times I found that he turned the stimulator on, and I would turn it off. Finally I took the stimulator away from him. I said, "This isn't helping you."

That evening, Braunwald was reviewing his patient's EKGs when he noticed something strange. When the stimulator was off, the patient had signs of severe ischemia, or impending heart attack, but when the patient turned it on—against Braunwald's explicit instructions—the EKG became "almost normal." "So he was right and I was wrong!" he mused. Braunwald compares a heart attack to a light switch. Until that time, in his analogy, doctors viewed a heart attack as causing immediate and permanent damage that could be neither limited nor reversed—much like a light switch that is flipped off. But what he learned from his wayward patient, and the fact that his EKG improved when the stimulator was turned on, was that ongoing damage from a heart attack *could* be limited. He concluded that maybe a heart attack was more "like a dimmer switch" that offered a window of time during which doctors could "resurrect" the heart.

Although Braunwald's electrical device would ultimately fail as a treatment for angina, it provided the conceptual basis for the VNS device that was implanted in Dennis Fegan to control his seizures. Cyberonics, the company that won a patent for this device, cited Braunwald's work in dozens of patent applications. The company wanted to use the device to treat not only seizures but also everything from depression and obesity to drug addiction, anxiety, hypertension, and hiccups.[77]

Once the device was on the market, many patients with seizures and their neurologists would praise it as miraculous. One caretaker of a patient implanted with a VNS device reported that any time the patient began to have a seizure, all he had to do was turn the device on, and the seizure would stop immediately. He said, "It works really well; it's like magic!"

Braunwald's discovery of the therapeutic power of vagus nerve stimulation—and the ability of a company like Cyberonics to harness that power in the form of a patented device—is a classic example of the innovative capabilities of the medical-industrial complex. Brilliant scientific insight, well-honed medical instincts, groundbreaking research, and the entrepreneurial quest for profit came together to produce a technological breakthrough that appeared to benefit many thousands of patients with a host of varied conditions.

Unfortunately, for many people like Dennis Fegan, the story doesn't end there.

Chapter Three

DEADLY DEVICES

FOR THE FIRST FEW months after Dennis Fegan had the VNS device implanted in his neck in 2000, he thought it was working well—a typical "honeymoon period," as he would later describe it. He was having somewhat fewer seizures, without any apparent side effects from the device. But slowly the seizures resumed, and soon they were just as frequent and as bad as ever. Even worse, he began to develop new symptoms. The first thing he noticed was a change in his "aura"—the visual, auditory, and tactile sensations that can herald the onset of seizures. In the past his auras had varied, in keeping with the variety of temporal seizures. Sometimes the aura would feel like a grain of sand flicking over his face. At other times he couldn't describe how he knew a fit was coming except to say that a certain feeling would come over him.

One thing was consistent, though: his auras had never been painful. But several years after he was implanted with the VNS device, he began to have a painful sensation in his throat right before his seizures hit. When the pain started, he knew he had only fifteen seconds before he'd lose consciousness. "I'd feel like I was choking. Then I'd cough, and the next thing I knew I'd pass out and wake up on the ground."

Along with the change in his aura, the period after his seizures changed. Normally, if he lost consciousness, he would have a typical after-seizure syndrome known as a postictal state, the hallmark of grand mal seizures. During the postictal state, he'd be profoundly tired, groggy, and confused. The symptoms would clear gradually over an hour or two. Now he was finding himself suddenly sprawled on the floor but wide awake, with no grogginess or confusion.

From his reading about epilepsy, he knew that a certain rare type of seizure, known as a drop or atonic seizure, could cause people to abruptly drop to the ground and recover almost immediately.[78] Such seizures are caused by a sudden break in the electrical impulses from brain to muscle, impulses that are necessary not only to spark muscles to contract but also to give them their tone, even at rest. Without these impulses, muscles abruptly stop working, and the affected individual simply goes limp, like a human rag doll, and drops to the floor, sometimes causing serious injuries. Occasionally, the only muscles affected might be in the head and neck, causing the eyelids to droop and the head to flop forward on the chest. Typically the episodes last from mere seconds to a minute or two, and the individual remains conscious.

Fegan told Bahamon about his new aura, the throat pain, and the drop seizures. He wasn't overly concerned when Bahamon didn't provide any insight or specific new treatment for his symptoms. As Fegan says, "I had lots of different types of seizures. That's what temporal lobe epilepsy is like. So I just figured I was having a new type of seizure."

But there was a puzzling aspect to his new seizures. Drop seizures are generally abrupt and give no warning. There is no aura, so the fact that Fegan was having what seemed to be a new type of aura consisting of throat pain and a cough before his seizures was mysterious. Another unusual development was that he *was* losing consciousness, which isn't common with drop seizures. These odd symptoms were pointing to something else entirely, but at the time, neither Fegan nor his neurologist had any idea what.

Finally, in late 2004 or early 2005, he'd had enough. Although Fegan could turn off the device temporarily with his magnet, he asked his neurologist to permanently disable the VNS with the programming wand. It wasn't preventing his seizures, he was still on a boatload of medicines, and he just wanted the damned thing turned off. Even though the VNS had been implanted more than four years earlier, his neurologist suggested that he give it more time. The manufacturer, Cyberonics, claimed it could take a year or two for the device to help. Maybe Fegan's was just taking longer to kick in.

In June of 2006, six years after the device was implanted, he had one of his new "drop attacks," taking a hard fall that crushed the bones in his left wrist. The surgeon said he'd have to wait for the swelling to go down before he could have surgery to insert a metal plate to hold the bones together.

About six weeks before the fall, he'd been started on Inderal, a medicine to treat tremors caused by his seizure meds. Inderal can slow the heart rate and lower blood pressure, especially at high doses. If the pulse or blood pressure drops far enough, it can cause light-headedness or fainting. But there was no evidence that the Inderal, which Fegan was taking in low doses, was causing his heart to slow or his blood pressure, which had been a bit high, to drop. And his drop attacks had started *before* he was placed on Inderal. So with nothing to suggest that the drug was causing a problem, his doctor continued Fegan on the medicine.

It was then, less than two weeks after his fall, and before his wrist surgery was scheduled, that Fegan's parents went to his house to drop off his egg-and-potato taquitos and found him, as we saw, in very bad shape, repeatedly losing consciousness, at which point he was taken by ambulance to Corpus Christi Medical Center.

Dr. Larry Johnson, the doctor on duty at the Corpus Christi Medical Center ER on Sunday morning, July 2, 2006, says he remembers Dennis Fegan more clearly than any other patient he has treated during his thirty years as an ER doctor.[79] When he first saw Fegan, he thought he was in status epilepticus—a state of continuous seizures. He had powerful drugs he could administer to stop the seizures, and the first-line drug for status is diazepam (Valium), which the paramedics had already given him intravenously. Despite the medicine, Fegan kept passing out. The outlook was not good.

While examining Fegan, Johnson looked up at the sound of an alarm and was startled by what he saw on Fegan's heart monitor: the steady blip-blip-blip of heartbeats scrolling across the monitor was followed by a long flat line, which had triggered the monitor's high-pitched wail. It was the sort of flat line shown on television dramas that signals that a patient has just died. Fegan was going into asystole (pronounced "a-SIS-toh-lee"), meaning that all the electrical activity of his heart was stopping. And it was stopping for so long that Fegan was passing out—not from seizures but from lack of oxygen to the brain.

Johnson recalls, "He would seem to be trying to clear his throat by coughing. Then he would become pale and unresponsive to any stimuli.... He was in complete asystole. I remember striking him on the chest to attempt to jolt his heart into beating again."

In television shows, patients are dramatically saved with a jolt to the chest, but in real life, even immediate emergency care by doctors rarely saves a patient whose heart has flatlined. And Fegan kept going back into asystole. Johnson recalls his fear that he was not going to be able to save this seemingly healthy man who was too young to die. Individuals with epilepsy are two to three times more likely than individuals in the general population to die early. Seizure-related deaths can result from status epilepticus or from a disorder known as sudden unexpected death in epilepsy (SUDEP), which tends to occur in the aftermath of a grand mal seizure, particularly in individuals whose seizures are poorly controlled.[80-83] Estimates of the rate of SUDEP vary widely, depending on a person's age and other factors, and the exact cause of SUDEP is uncertain. Experts theorize that it could be caused by sudden cessation of breathing or heartbeat caused by deranged brain function. Had Fegan died that day, as it seemed likely he would, Johnson might very well have cited SUDEP as the probable cause, not knowing how else to explain the heart stoppages. Luckily, as Johnson watched Fegan's heart monitor, he noticed a curious thing: Fegan was lapsing into asystole at precise three-minute intervals. Johnson didn't know anything about Fegan, his history, or about the VNS device implanted in his chest. Emergency doctors don't have the privilege of learning about patients in critical condition before they treat them. Serious injuries from car crashes, gunshot wounds, and knife wounds have to be treated. Hemorrhages have to be stopped. And hearts that aren't beating must be restarted.

Johnson called in a cardiologist who came to the ER. Fegan's neurologist, alerted by his family, was on his way as well. All three doctors stood watching the monitor, and all witnessed the strange phenomenon: every three minutes, Fegan's heart flatlined. As the doctors conferred, something Bahamon told them made the diagnosis clear: Fegan's VNS device was set to fire at three-minute intervals.

The doctors came to a sudden, startling conclusion. What had looked like seizures was actually a side effect of Fegan's VNS device.

One of the main functions of the vagus nerve is to slow the heart rate. Now the device was doing its job with deadly efficiency: each time the VNS fired, it was not just slowing Fegan's heart rate, it was also causing his heart to stop altogether. The VNS had to be turned off—and *fast*. It was impossible to tell how much longer Fegan could withstand the episodes of asystole.

Bahamon was unprepared for this new diagnosis. When Fegan's parents called him, he was told Fegan was having seizures. He didn't suspect a problem with the device and didn't bring the programming wand to turn it off. Wanting to stay with his patient, he turned to Fegan's mother, who'd arrived minutes earlier. Could she run to her son's home to get Fegan's magnet? The magnet, used to activate the VNS, couldn't turn the device off permanently, but it could disable it temporarily. Irene raced out of the ER and headed back to her son's house.

When Fegan was brought in by the ambulance crew, Johnson had immediately ordered blood tests, drug levels, and a twelve-lead EKG. The tests would tell him if Fegan had suffered a heart attack or had liver, kidney, or thyroid dysfunction. Now the results were coming back. Fegan's complete blood count and electrolytes were normal. The level of valproic acid (a medicine to treat seizures) in his blood was in the therapeutic (correct) range. His blood oxygen level was normal. With no underlying problem to treat, there was nothing else to do.

Johnson recalls the tense vigil as the doctors waited for Fegan's mother to return with the magnet. The minutes ticked by. They watched helplessly as Fegan continued to lose consciousness and Johnson continued to attempt resuscitation, knowing that with each new episode of asystole, Fegan's chance of survival was becoming vanishingly small. Finally the wait grew to be too much for Bahamon. He decided to risk leaving his patient's bedside and raced back to his office to retrieve his own wand. When he returned to the ER, Johnson was still doing everything in his power to keep Fegan alive. Bahamon took out the wand, pressed it against Fegan's chest, and within a minute, the device was off. Fegan's "seizures" and asystole immediately stopped. Once the doctors realized that his heart was beating normally and their patient was safe, Johnson had him moved to the hospital's intensive care unit to recover. All three doctors documented the link between Fegan's asystole and the VNS device, indicating that his "seizures" stopped as soon as the device was deactivated. Fegan would have no further episodes of asystole.

Fegan doesn't recall much about the day he was brought to the ER. Nor does he remember Johnson striking his chest in an attempt to get his heart restarted. But he does recall waking up in the intensive care unit and learning something that left him puzzled. "I saw someone standing at my bedside staring at my heart monitor," he says. "I didn't know who I was talking to, but I knew he was a doctor. I asked if I had a seizure, and he said no. So I asked what happened, and he said I had 'heart stoppages.' I didn't know if I heard him right. I said, 'Heart seizures?' And he said, 'No. Heart stoppages.' Then he introduced himself and told me he was a cardiologist. I was surprised because I knew I'd never had heart problems."

Fegan didn't learn why he'd had the "heart stoppages" until a day later, when Bahamon came to see him. "He told me that he had to go to his office to get the equipment to disable the vagus nerve stimulator, and once he did that [the "seizures"] stopped. He told me he just got off the phone with Cyberonics. He said he told them he was going to report what happened to the FDA." The FDA is the US government agency charged with regulating the manufacture and sale of medical devices.

When Fegan realized that the device in his chest had nearly killed him, he was confused. He thought back to his earlier seizures. They had started to change between six months to a year earlier, and he had told Bahamon about his new symptoms. How many times had he thought he was having seizures when it was really the device making his heart stop? How long had his "cure" been putting his life in danger?

Unbeknownst to Fegan or his doctors, his hospitalization for asystole would prove to be just the beginning of a downward spiral that would culminate in a horrifying and very public event.

* * *

Dr. Eugene Braunwald's 1967 experiment with electrical stimulation of the vagus nerve was the scientific breakthrough that would lead decades later to the implantation of Cyberonics' VNS device in Dennis Fegan's neck. But that connection would never have occurred without the complex web of scientific, economic, social, and political trends that, taken together, tell the story of the rise of the medical-industrial complex in the post–World War II US. Those interlocking interests would continue to ensnare Fegan again and again, long after he was hospitalized with "heart stoppages" in 2006. And it was that same web that would ultimately lead to Fegan's unraveling years later.

Three historical developments lie at the center of the rise of the medical-industrial complex: the explosion of medical technology beginning in the 1960s; the passage of Medicare in 1965, along with the proliferation of private health insurance; and the Bayh-Dole Act of 1980. Together these three developments drove the corporatization of medicine, with profound implications for the way healthcare is promoted, practiced, and regulated in the US.

The first development in this triad was the availability of new technologies that began to pour onto the market, such as bone-marrow transplants and cardiopulmonary bypass machines. But with new technologies came medical price tags beyond the reach of the average citizen. Prior to the mid-twentieth century, few US citizens had health insurance. Nor did they need it, in most instances. In the early 1900s, patients paid their doctors with a few dollars or by barter, with gifts of, say, chickens, or occasionally by performing a chore.[84] Hospital care was cheap, since hospitals had little to offer besides beds to rest in, nurses who could watch over patients following a heart attack, and maybe cheap antibiotics for the treatment of pneumonia. The primary expense of being sick wasn't medical care, it was loss of income.[85] A 1919 state of Illinois study found that lost wages cost workers four times as much as their medical expenses did.[86]

At the time, it was not uncommon for doctors to supplement their income as farmers or pharmacists. Although doctors' incomes rose to $5,000 ($68,000 in 2015 dollars) by 1929, their pay was still relatively modest: a quarter of doctors in 1929 earned less than $2,300. To put that in context, the average income in the US at this time was $1,800, and a train engineer could earn $4,700.[87]

Health insurance was first offered in the 1930s, mostly to cover hospital care.[86] It spread slowly. As recently as 1940, just 3 percent of the US population had health insurance. Outpatient coverage came even later. In 1950, only 12 percent of all healthcare costs were covered by insurance, and total costs for a doctor's visit remained low, at just three to five dollars per visit ($26 to $44 in 2015 dollars).[88] Millionaire doctors were yet to be minted: the average doctor in 1940 was still solidly middle class, earning just over twice the income of an average worker. By 1949, the average doctor earned $11,058, and the median family income was $3,400.[89]

Then, in the 1960s, researchers such as Eugene Braunwald began to take advantage of advances in electronics, computers, and biotechnology to invent new procedures, devices, and drugs. Over the subsequent few decades, during the "golden age" of medicine, new medical technologies poured onto the market. Medicine was transformed by CAT scans, MRIs, and PET scans, which could make visible every millimeter of the human body. The market was flooded with new implantable devices, including cardiac stents, designed to open blocked coronary arteries; cochlear implants, which could help deaf people hear; implantable cardioverter defibrillators, which could correct dangerous heart rhythms; and deep-brain stimulators, to help people with Parkinson's disease. But these technologies came with eye-popping price tags that only a handful of wealthy individuals could afford.

Medicare would change all that.

This second historical development was set in motion in 1965, when President Lyndon Johnson signed Medicare into law. Medicare served two main political and economic purposes; it provided a hedge against growing demand for a national health program by offering coverage to seniors rather than the entire population. It also opened up a vast new market for costly healthcare technologies, transforming senior citizens, regardless of their personal financial circumstances, into relatively affluent medical consumers.

Initially, the American Medical Association (AMA), representing US physicians, had vigorously opposed Medicare as "socialized medicine."[90] As passage of the law became increasingly unavoidable, lobbyists for the AMA, which contributed campaign money to politicians, pressured Congress and won several concessions to ensure that doctors would get a big cut of the goodies. Paul Starr, author of the Pulitzer Prize–winning book *The Social Transformation of Medicine,* tracks the role the AMA played in shaping Medicare for the financial benefit of doctors.[91] The provisions inserted into Medicare by the AMA delivered more than one Trojan horse to the public.

In her book *Overtreated: Why Too Much Medicine Is Making Us Sicker and Poorer,* Shannon Brownlee, senior vice president of the Lown Institute, in Brookline, Massachusetts, explains the complex, far-reaching impact of the advent of Medicare on the US healthcare system. Some of the results, she notes, were unquestionably positive: "One of the great social programs of the twentieth century, Medicare not only made healthcare available to millions of elderly citizens, it also spurred the desegregation of hospitals in the South— and brought down infant mortality rates among African Americans as a result." But not all the changes Medicare effected were for the public good. "For all their worries about socialized medicine imperiling their livelihoods," Brownlee says, doctors would in the end "reap a bonanza from Medicare."[90]

One AMA provision ensured that doctors would be paid on a fee-for-service basis for whatever they said was their "usual and customary" fee. This created a bonanza for doctors and led to dramatic increases in prices for healthcare services. Fee-for-service payments provided financial incentives for doctors to do more things to patients because they were paid more for doing more. More tests. More surgeries. More procedures. More pills. Of course, this incentive had always been there, but now the scale was several orders of magnitude greater. Since doctors could bill Medicare at far higher prices than they could reasonably expect the average patient to pay out of pocket, doctors began to claim ever-escalating "usual and customary" fees. Conversely, the kinds of nonquantifiable, impossible-to-charge-for services that patients often need and want most, such as the availability of a doctor who will spend time listening to them and carefully discussing options, were not rewarded by the Medicare system.

Another feature of Medicare that contributed to the spectacular rise in national healthcare expenditures was that it specifically excluded a cap on payments.[90, 91] Unlike a single-payer system, in which government budgets a certain amount of money for healthcare, just as it does for defense, education, and policing, Medicare was infinitely expandable. Whatever doctors charged and no matter how often they submitted charges, Medicare paid.[91]

Although some changes in reimbursement schemes for Medicare payments, including price caps, would be instituted many years later, the initial cap exclusion opened the door to soaring profits for doctors and hospitals. Routine hospital, intensive-care unit, and coronary-care unit stays costing tens and even hundreds of thousands of dollars were now possible. Suddenly healthcare prices were soaring far beyond what the average Joe or Jane without Medicare could afford. This in turn led to a surge in demand for private and worker-based health insurance, because those without Medicare could no longer afford medical treatment. By 1986, just twenty years after the passage of Medicare, fully 84 percent of the population was covered by health insurance.[92]

Another provision of Medicare resulted in cost-plus payments to hospitals, i.e., whatever price hospitals set as their "costs" would be reimbursed by the government with an additional fee on top, which also ensured a rising price tag, because hospitals were paid more if they charged more. Brownlee has bemoaned the arrangement, saying it allowed hospitals to make out "just like the Beltway bandit military suppliers."

Because the demand for hospitalization is largely under the control of doctors, admission rates don't necessarily reflect the needs of patients but often are driven by hospitals' financial need to fill their beds. As a result, cost-plus payments meant that hospital charges rose at a spectacular rate. Brownlee describes the financial cycle this way: "Build a new wing, fill it up, your costs rise, and therefore your reimbursements and profits rise. Build build build! And of course you need more hospital-based nursing and physician labor to staff all those beds, and so our hospital-centric system grew and grew and grew—at the expense of community and home-based care. House calls went the way of the bleeding cup and the leech."[90]

The evolving economic system affected healthcare in other ways, many of them unpredictable. With the rise of multiple insurers, doctors had to deal with endless insurance forms as well as the varying standards of care required by third parties. Consequently, administrative costs began to soar until they came to consume about 20 percent of healthcare expenditures. This led many doctors to sell their practices to large practice groups that could handle the flood of paperwork. Banding together into groups also allowed doctors to pool the capital resources needed to pay for expensive equipment, such as CT scanners, which in 2012 had an average list price of $1.2 million.[93]

Over time, many doctors became disenchanted with practice groups and their incessant meetings and disagreements about how to handle the business side of medicine, leading many doctors to agree to sign on as employees of large groups or hospitals that span entire towns, states, and, in some instances, nations. Thus the long-term impact of Medicare was both a vast expansion of national spending on healthcare services and the transformation of healthcare from a cottage industry made up of thousands of small independent providers to a corporatized business dominated by big companies.

The third key development was the Bayh-Dole Act, passed in 1980. This law, intended to promote innovation through "technology transfer," allowed public universities to patent the products of their research for the first time. Bayh-Dole institutionalized financial incentives that encouraged scientific researchers at universities to focus more on discoveries with major commercial potential than on those with long-term, purely scientific, or public-health value.[94] The monetary incentives set in motion by Bayh-Dole have led to a number of scandals involving falsified, exaggerated, or distorted medical research claims (more on those scandals later).

Thanks in large part to these three factors—the rise of technologically based medical care, the passage of Medicare along with the rise of private health insurance, and the Bayh-Dole Act, which rewarded commercial research at universities—the medical-industrial complex was born. It is a behemoth made up of interlocking organizational interests: hospitals, insurers, professional medical associations, pharmaceuticals companies, device manufacturers, research institutions, medical journals, electronic-medical-record developers, and many more. All these parties are economically dependent, ultimately, on the existence of end products for sale: medical treatments, drugs, surgeries, and devices, from insulin to pacemakers to life-support machines. Without those products, many of the insurers, the hospitals, the manufacturers, and even the doctors themselves would have no market, no income, and no reason for existing. Thus the logic of the marketplace makes it all but inevitable that this network of interested individuals and organizations must, consciously or unconsciously, devote much of its time, energy, and financial resources to promoting more sales of its products—more drugs, more medical procedures, more tests, more surgeries, more medical devices, and so on.

From the 1960s through 1980, advocates of free-market healthcare supported each of these developments on the grounds that market forces increase efficiency and put downward pressure on spending. Those predictions proved wrong. In 1950, US health expenditures accounted for just 4.6 percent of the gross domestic product. By 2009, they consumed 17 percent of the GDP.[87, 95] Healthcare spending continued to accelerate from there, and by 2015 expenditures reached $3.2 trillion. One of every five dollars in the US now goes to pay for medical expenses.

Today, for the first time in history, instead of being compensated as teachers and engineers are, it's possible for doctors, hospital CEOs, and insurance executives to become multimillionaires. In a capitalist society like the one in the US, the availability of unlimited profits is a powerful motivating force. The vast sums of money that began to pour into healthcare in the late 1960s inevitably attracted big corporations, ambitious entrepreneurs, and savvy investors looking for profitable opportunities. And just as inevitably, they began to influence the motivations and expectations of healthcare providers, even people who'd originally entered the field for noble humanitarian reasons. Companies and their employees may be forced to adopt the same ethically questionable methods and incentives their competitors use, lest they fail in the marketplace, making it difficult for even the most well-intentioned people to act in ways consistent with their values. And for some individuals, seeing colleagues and industry rivals becoming wealthy doing the same kind of work as they do, can encourage the choice to get in on the action.

One of the most powerful and rapidly growing participants in this burgeoning economic network is the medical device industry. Generating estimated revenues of more than $136 billion in the US in 2014, the implantable-device industry is even more lucrative for many of its component companies than the highly profitable pharmaceuticals industry.[96, 97] Operating-profit margins for the largest companies include 30.0 percent for Zimmer Biomet (artificial joints), 28.6 percent for Medtronic, 25.8 percent for St. Jude Medical, and 23.1 percent for Stryker (orthopedic implants).[97] Johnson & Johnson's device division squirreled away $7.2 billion in profits in 2012, while Medtronic pulled down $3.6 billion in profits that year.[98] Ultra-high prices help fuel those giant profit margins: Medtronic charges approximately $19,000 for a neurostimulator used to treat back pain, which is four times what it costs to manufacture the device. Hospitals pay $4,500–$7,500 for a popular type of hip implant that costs $350 to manufacture.[98] Hospitals are asked to sign confidentiality agreements, obliging them not to reveal their purchase prices.

Implantable devices have become fixtures of the healthcare landscape. No one knows how many millions of Americans are walking around today with medical devices implanted in their bodies. Unlike drugs, which are labeled, dated, and tracked, there is no comparable tracking system for medical devices. An effort to correct the problem with unique device identifiers (UDIs) has been under way for well over a decade, and although most devices will have to have bar codes by 2020 indicating the UDI, there is currently no mechanism or requirement to incorporate the UDIs in patients' electronic health records, thus undermining their central purposes: to allow tracking of device performance and to rapidly notify implanted patients of device problems or recalls.[99, 100]

Millions of Americans are implanted with devices annually: half a million have stents placed in their coronary arteries each year, while nearly a million have artificial hips, knees, and shoulders implanted. In 2002, one expert calculated that one of every ten Americans is implanted with a medical device. If the 10 percent rate of 2002 holds true today, that would mean that thirty-two million Americans have implanted devices in their bodies and are profoundly affected (for better or worse) by the way the FDA approves, monitors, and manages those devices. With the rapid increase of implantable devices in the past decade, however, the number of Americans with an implanted device is probably substantially more than thirty-two million. A 2011 review found that 6.7 million individuals were implanted annually with the top eleven implanted devices—meaning that in just over ten years, some seventy million individuals were implanted. And of course, as profit-seeking corporations, device makers use a portion of their huge profits to mount marketing and advertising campaigns designed to convince doctors and ordinary citizens that even more medical devices are needed.

The allure and remarkable benefit of some devices is undeniable. John Calhoun, a sixty-four-year-old man with a pacemaker, says he's delighted to have the device inside him. "I have to take pills every day for my high blood pressure, and it reminds me every day that I have a problem. Besides, it's a hassle. But the pacemaker is just there." He taps the spot under his collarbone where a small bulge gives away the presence of the pacemaker. "I don't have to think about it. And it's saved my life."

Certain devices have changed many lives for the better. Artificial lenses used in cataract surgery have restored vision to millions who would otherwise have been functionally blind. Pacemakers keep hearts beating. And artificial hip joints have allowed previously bedridden and wheelchair-bound patients to walk again.

But sadly, countless patients have also been betrayed by the companies that manufactured the devices implanted in their bodies and by the regulatory authorities that were supposed to ensure that these devices would help rather than harm them. And just as we don't know how many people are currently implanted with medical devices, we don't know how many people die each year from complications caused by medical devices. An estimate by the Brookings Institution pegged the number at three thousand.[101] But the actual number could be much higher. In 2015, approximately sixteen thousand deaths associated with medical devices were reported to the FDA. And a Government Accountability Office analysis found that *99 percent of device-related "adverse events" are never reported to the FDA* and that the "more serious the event, the less likely it was to be reported."[102] Based on the GAO analysis, that means medical devices could have been associated with as many as 1.6 million deaths in 2015. Even if only 1 to 10 percent of those deaths were *caused* by a device, that means between 16,000 and 160,000 people may have been killed by devices, making medical devices one of the leading causes of death in the US.

So why is the Brookings estimate three thousand while the FDA's own database reveals approximately sixteen thousand *reported* deaths in 2015? It's a mystery. The Brookings report was produced under a cooperative agreement between the FDA and the Engelberg Center for Healthcare Reform at the Brookings Institution. Former and current FDA experts, including former FDA commissioner Mark McClellan, authored the report, which according to Brookings took a good deal of expertise and "countless hours" of research to compile. But neither the FDA nor Brookings was able to explain how they arrived at the estimate of three thousand deaths, which was reported by the *New York Times, Modern Healthcare,* and other outlets.

In an e-mail to me dated August 29, 2016, a spokesperson for the FDA stated, "The report does not provide a citation for its mention of the 50,000 serious injuries and 3,000 deaths, so it is unclear how these numbers were derived."

Brookings is funded in part by drug and device manufacturers (for example, in 2015, Genentech, which develops both drugs and devices, contributed between $500,000 and $999,999 to Brookings). The planning board for the report included representatives of device makers such as Medtronic, United BioSource, and ReVision Optics. Conspicuously absent from the planning board were members of any watchdog groups, such as the Public Citizen Health Research Group or the National Center for Health Research, among others.[101]

The truth about the number of deaths caused by medical devices is that it is unknown. There is simply no way to arrive at a reliable estimate, because no one is keeping track. Not the FDA. Not the manufacturers. Not professional or trade societies. Not hospitals. Not doctors.

Since no one knows for sure how many people have medical devices in their bodies or how many people are injured or die from implanted medical devices, their impact is not at all clear. This might seem deeply disturbing—because it is. Especially because the technology to know isn't lacking: Walmart tracks every single head of lettuce it buys and sells and can determine how many heads of lettuce are on its shelves at any given moment, yet no one—not the FDA, not Brookings, not anyone—can say how many people are dying because of implanted medical devices. It's a black hole.

Complicating our understanding of implanted devices, which can be even more dangerous than prescribed drugs, are some widespread misperceptions.

First, most of us assume that if a medical device is on the market, there must be evidence that the FDA has vetted it as safe and effective. In fact, for most devices, this is not the case. While there has been a good deal of criticism about the FDA's failure to protect the public from drugs that are unsafe or ineffective, drug manufacturers are at least supposed to prove the value of their products in one and generally two clinical trials. What the public and many doctors don't realize is that the same is not true for even the highest-risk implanted devices. Despite claims by the FDA that high-risk implanted medical devices have to undergo "rigorous premarket testing," the agency requires clinical testing for only a small fraction of high-risk devices. Indeed, according to a 2009 study published in the *Journal of the American Medical Association*, only five percent of the highest-risk cardiac devices have undergone the sort of testing that comes even close to the testing required for drug approvals.[15]* Even when devices are subjected to clinical testing, the quality of the studies performed is frequently poor, producing unreliable information.[13, 14, 15]

Another common misperception is that devices are inert objects and therefore do not have side effects, as drugs do. Device manufacturers often play on this assumption, suggesting in promotional materials that patients can use devices to treat everything from epilepsy to Parkinson's and coronary heart disease "without drug side effects." Sure, if you get implanted with a medical device you won't need to worry about the side effects of drugs *if* you are no longer taking them. However, patients often must keep taking drugs even after implantation with a device. Test subjects given the VNS device for epilepsy, for example, continued taking their seizure medicines. And for some devices, patients have to take *more* drugs in order for their device to function safely.

Then there's the array of side effects and complications caused

---

* For more on how devices are approved by the FDA, see Chapter Six.

by devices that can be even more deadly than drugs. But brochures for medical devices often bury that information in the small print or leave it out altogether.

One study found that of 113 device recalls initiated because of a risk of serious injury or death, only 19 percent had been approved through the PMA process,* meaning that 81 percent of devices that caused the worst harm were cleared or approved through pathways that didn't require clinical testing by the FDA.[103]

To make matters worse, doctors are often unfamiliar with or even unaware of the existence of implanted devices in their patients and the side effects they cause, making it impossible to correctly identify certain problems and take remedial action.

Unlike drugs, implanted devices require surgery, which carries its own risks, including bleeding, infection, organ perforation, complications from anesthesia, and other mishaps. Even devices that can be injected, such as certain filters intended to trap blood clots or stents placed in coronary arteries, involve invasive procedures or surgery that entails certain risks. Arteries can be (and have been) sheared during cardiac catheterizations performed to implant stents, causing massive bleeding, shock, heart attack, multiorgan failure, and death.

Many devices present two unique and potentially serious problems: first, patients implanted with certain metallic devices cannot have an MRI scan because the strong magnetic field could cause the device to move and tear the flesh or heat up and cause burns.[104, 105] Reports in the FDA database reveal that patients implanted with the VNS device have been burned, causing extreme pain, and the June 2014 patient manual for the device states that

---

* The exact percentage of devices for which clinical data were submitted is uncertain; only 16 to 19 percent of all high-risk devices go through the PMA approval process. The only other pathway requiring testing data is one of four supplemental pathways, which was found to comprise only 0.3 percent of all approvals. No information is available on testing data submitted for that pathway.

even after it is removed, if as little as an inch of lead wire remains implanted, the result can be "serious injury (e.g., burn of the vagus nerve and surrounding tissue)." Implanted devices such as breast implants can also cause opacity or distortions on imaging that prevent diagnosis of problems, such as cancer. The FDA cautions that CAT scans can interfere with the functioning of certain "insulin pumps, cardiac implantable electronic devices, and neurostimulators."

Computerized devices are potentially subject to hackers.[106] A seemingly fanciful episode of the Showtime television series *Homeland* features assassins killing the vice president by hacking his pacemaker and disabling it. The capability of hackers to cause deadly harm is so real that Vice President Dick Cheney's cardiologist, Jonathan Reiner of George Washington University Hospital, in Washington, DC, disabled the wireless feature on Cheney's pacemaker, saying, "It seemed to me to be a bad idea for the vice president to have a device that maybe somebody on a rope line or in the next hotel room or downstairs might be able to get into—hack into."[107]

The computer security expert Barnaby Jack demonstrated that he could remotely hack devices, causing insulin pumps to deliver lethal doses of insulin and triggering pacemaker-defibrillators to deliver 830-volt shocks to a patient.[108] Jack, who died the day before he was to reveal how he accomplished the hacks, said he was working with the manufacturers to secure the devices.[109] Despite Jack's white-hat attempts to spur action, the problem remains. In 2017, experts warned that some thirty-six thousand medical devices are "easily discoverable."[110] And others have said that many devices are vulnerable to malicious computer worms that could cause "mass murder." Although such actions seem unlikely, it's worrisome that the engineers and hackers who are demonstrating these vulnerabilities may have a parallel in the engineers who warned, years in advance of Hurricane Katrina, that the levees of New Orleans were at risk.

And pacemakers aren't the only computerized devices that use Bluetooth technology and Wi-Fi connectivity to allow doctors to monitor and manage patients' devices from many miles away. Millions of Americans are implanted with deep-brain stimulators, cardiac defibrillators, gastric stimulators, insulin pumps, foot-drop implants, cochlear implants, and the VNS, which are all potential targets for hackers—in part because the FDA has never required device makers to encrypt the data transmitted by the devices.[106, 111, 112] And, the experts warn, encryption is merely the first step necessary to protect the public.

In September of 2016, Jeffrey Shuren, director of FDA's Center for Devices and Radiological Health, signed a memorandum of understanding with various stakeholders, including Homeland Security, law enforcement, and intelligence agencies, encouraging "identification, mitigation, and prevention of cybersecurity threats to medical devices."[111]

Individuals implanted with devices, whether computerized or not, have yet another problem: turning off or removing a device is not as easy as discontinuing a drug. Patients can be weaned off even the most dangerous or addictive drugs, but many electrical devices, such as pacemakers, defibrillators, and nerve stimulators, continue to cause pain and harm while attempts are made to turn them off, and some implanted devices are extremely difficult to remove. Material from pacemakers and VNS devices often becomes embedded in human tissue, causing scar formation that traps lead wires, mesh, and tubing and making removal a dangerous and sometimes fatal endeavor. When Medtronic recalled Sprint Fidelis defibrillator leads, many patients rushed to have them removed, but removal posed its own dangers, causing major complications in 15.3 percent of patients.[113] The most recent "upgraded" models presented the greatest risk, with a complication rate of 18.7 percent.

There are other sharp differences between drugs and devices that should be considered before anyone agrees to an implant. For individuals with serious problems, such as vision loss and heart-rhythm disturbances, implantable devices can be transformative and livesaving. But without adequate information about the efficacy and safety of the vast majority of devices, from spine implants to stents and surgical mesh, many citizens are being treated worse than guinea pigs. At least the results of experiments performed on guinea pigs are monitored to observe the value of an intervention, whereas postsurgical monitoring of humans implanted with devices is often nonexistent. Although the FDA is awash in monitoring programs, the reality is that they are largely ineffective, and without adequate preapproval testing, and without ongoing monitoring and enforcement by the FDA of requirements for postapproval safety studies, there is simply no certainty about the likelihood of an individual being helped or harmed by a device.

For all these reasons, the medical device industry is one of the most powerful yet unaccountable sectors of the medical-industrial complex. Fegan's discovery that his supposedly lifesaving VNS device had almost killed him would also prove to be just the first in a series of revelations about how great a danger device makers pose to the health of millions of Americans.

Chapter Four

THE MAN FROM CYBERONICS

IN AUGUST OF 2006, one month after he was discharged from the hospital, Dennis Fegan was recovering at home when he received a phone call from Dr. Juan Bahamon's office. A secretary told him that a representative from Cyberonics was on the other line. The representative wanted to speak with him. Would he...She couldn't finish her sentence before he shouted, "They nearly killed me! Why would I want to talk with them?" and slammed the phone down.

A few weeks later, he learned that Cyberonics had made another call. This time they asked to have a company representative present during Fegan's next appointment with Bahamon. The neurologist agreed. By the time Fegan was informed that the Cyberonics representative would attend his one-month follow-up, he had begun to cool off. He began to think about why the company might want to meet with him. Since he believed that Bahamon had always looked out for his best interests and had agreed to the meeting, he reasoned that perhaps the company was going to offer him money. Maybe lots of money! Money to shut him up. After all, he'd been telling everyone he knew about what the VNS device had done to him.

He recalls the meeting with a bitter laugh: "If they offered me a check for a couple hundred thousand dollars I might have taken it." But offering Fegan money was not what Cyberonics had in mind. Fegan says,

> Dr. Bahamon and I were in the office for just a few minutes before the Cyberonics rep came in. He was young and well dressed. The first question Bahamon asked him was, 'Are you a doctor?' The rep said no, but that he was trained to read EKGs. All I remember is him looking at my ER report and looking at the [heart monitor] strips. He didn't ask me any questions. It seemed like I was there just as a spectator. Then he asked Bahamon to perform a lead test. I could tell that Bahamon was uneasy to begin with, but when the rep asked him to do a lead test, he became angry. He raised his voice and said he wouldn't think of doing something like that unless I was in the hospital.

Fegan remembers a couple of other details from his encounter with the Cyberonics representative, Steven Parnis. He asked Parnis (whose title was senior manager of clinical engineering) whether Cyberonics planned to report his "incident" to the FDA. Fegan says Parnis "danced around" an answer, failing to commit one way or the other. He also remembers Parnis telling him and Bahamon that the company hadn't seen other cases like his. In fact, he insisted that Fegan's experience was an isolated occurrence and pointedly suggested that if Fegan hadn't begun taking the blood pressure and tremor-reducing drug Inderal, perhaps his heart wouldn't have stopped.

The meeting ended abruptly and without any discussion of

compensation. Fegan, hesitant to speak up, didn't ask any other questions of either Parnis or his doctor. He left feeling puzzled more than anything else.

When he got home, he looked up "lead test" on his computer. Even when he learned that the VNS device would have to be turned back on to do a lead test, it took a while for the implications to sink in. When they did, he grew angry: Cyberonics was asking his doctor to turn the device back on. The device Fegan wanted out of his body. The device that had almost killed him and that could kill him if it was reactivated.

His indignation mounted into a slow-burning fury that roiled his insides and fueled many late nights as he sat in the dark bedroom he'd turned into an office, searching the Internet to learn everything he could about the vagus nerve stimulator. He quickly learned that stimulation of the vagus nerve slows the heart rate. It seemed all too plausible that stimulation with an electrical device could slow the heart rate too much—even stop it.

Shortly after the visit from the Cyberonics senior manager, Fegan received a letter from Bahamon stating that he could no longer care for Fegan; he had thirty days to find another neurologist.[114] Bahamon didn't give a reason for dismissing Fegan from his patient roster; presumably he was fearful that Fegan might sue him. But Fegan believed that Bahamon had saved his life when he raced back to his office to get his programming wand so he could turn off the device, and he was disappointed to lose his long-term neurologist. He never did file a suit or a complaint against Bahamon and still doesn't fault him for referring him to a surgeon for the VNS implant. Fegan believes that Bahamon was a victim of Cyberonics' claims, just as he was. He concedes that maybe Bahamon could have looked into the device's track record further, but after all, the doctor was only trying to help him when he made the recommendation.

To this day, Dennis Fegan is reluctant to find fault with any of the physicians who cared for him. And perhaps he is right. There is plenty of blame to go around and no shortage of others who played a role in Fegan's long ordeal.

★ ★ ★

If Dr. Juan Bahamon was merely a bit player in the story of Dennis Fegan's near-death experience, what about Cyberonics, the company that had developed, designed, built, and marketed the deadly device?

Few physicians and even fewer patients know the history of Cyberonics,[*] despite the fact that approximately seventy-five thousand people with epilepsy have been persuaded to bet their lives on the quality of its product. The story of the company is a fascinating example of how the intertwined forces of scientific exploration, medical need, government regulation, and good old-fashioned capitalist greed are now shaping the American healthcare system, for good or ill. And it's a story that takes us back to the pioneering work of Dr. Eugene Braunwald.

The vagus nerve is one of the most remarkable components of the human body. It is the longest nerve in the autonomic nervous system, winding from the brain down through the neck, chest, abdomen, and pelvis and sending off branches to almost all the body's major organs. This means that stimulation of the vagus can produce an amazing variety of results—including slowing the heart rate, aiding digestion, and promoting orgasm.

According to the late emergency physician and Harvard Medical School alumnus Francis Fesmire, stimulating the vagus nerve can even cure hiccups—no laughing matter when they persist for days,

---

[*] In a $2.7 billion merger in October of 2015, Cyberonics joined with the Sorin Group to become LivaNova, which now sells the VNS device.

weeks, and even months, an exhausting affair that makes patients and their doctors grow desperate for a cure. And Fesmire found one. In 1988, he discovered that wiggling a finger in the rectum of a patient plagued with intractable hiccups made the problem vanish. The reason: the vagus nerve stimulates the diaphragm, the huge plate-like muscle at the floor of the lungs, which regulates breathing. When electrical impulses to the diaphragm go haywire, they can cause spasmodic contractions of the muscle, resulting in hiccups. Fesmire reasoned that digitally stimulating the terminal branch of the vagus nerve in the rectum could reset the electrical impulses and stop the spasms. Of course, no self-respecting academic would dream of announcing such a discovery in plain language. So he published his findings in *Annals of Emergency Medicine* under the title "Termination of Intractable Hiccups with Digital Rectal Massage," a publication that eighteen years later would win him one of the notorious Ig Nobel Prizes, presented at an annual ceremony at Harvard's Sanders Theatre. Author and musician Amanda Palmer has described the ceremony in her 2012 blog post, "Prizes for silly science: Ig Nobels tonight" on *Ready or Not, Here Come Science,* as "a collection of, like, actual Nobel Prize winners giving away prizes to real scientists for doing fucked-up things...it's awesome."

As Fesmire concluded his acceptance speech at the 2006 ceremony, the audience erupted in laughter when he displayed "Dr. Fran's Anti-Hiccup Kit" and announced that he was giving away a couple of dozen of them. Each contained just three items: a three-by-five-inch instruction card that displayed a picture of Fesmire, a latex glove, and a packet of lubricant.

In 1967, Eugene Braunwald discovered that stimulating the vagus nerve could be put to other uses. He knew that stimulating the vagus slows the heart rate, dilates blood vessels, and reduces the force of the heart's contractions, effects he believed could reduce heart pain, or angina pectoris. It was this theory that led Braunwald to implant the first VNS device in humans that same year and to describe in the prestigious *New England Journal of Medicine* the "striking improvement" in the first two patients he treated for angina by stimulating the carotid sinus (which cause vagus nerve stimulation).[115]

In 1970, Braunwald reported in the *Western Journal of Medicine* that early results of the treatment were "sufficiently encouraging to warrant continued trials of this new mode of therapy."[116] But buried in that report was a brief mention of a detail not included in either his conclusion or his later statements about the research: two of the first four patients had died in the immediate postoperative period—one from a heart attack caused by a critical slowing of the heart rate and the other from a drop in blood pressure. Both effects were known results of vagus nerve stimulation.

It's clear that Braunwald was not unaware of the risks of the device. Even in his original 1967 paper, he'd noted several potential dangers of vagus nerve stimulation, including nerve damage, "cardiac standstill or other dangerous arrhythmias," and the perils present in any surgical intervention. But in his later discussions of the VNS device, he offered few if any cautions about its potential dangers.

Braunwald's discovery was rapidly supplanted by coronary artery bypass surgery for coronary heart disease. So in time, Braunwald abandoned his work with the stimulator. But the papers published by this widely admired researcher about the potential of the VNS device remained in the medical literature, waiting to be rediscovered by some other ambitious scientist.

The moment came in the 1980s, when Jacob Zabara, PhD, a neurophysiologist at Temple University, speculated that stimulating the vagus nerve might interrupt seizures.[117] Zabara says the idea occurred to him when he saw his wife using breathing techniques to control labor pains during a Lamaze class. He wondered about the mechanism of pain control. Until this time, doctors thought the vagus nerve carried signals only away from the brain, not to it. Zabara wondered whether it was possible that the vagus nerve, which stimulates the diaphragm in breathing, might be sending information up to the brain and in some way regulating pain. And if the nerve could control pain, might it also control seizures or nausea if stimulated?

Although his line of reasoning isn't exactly clear, Zabara filed for a patent on the vagus nerve stimulator. In his patent application, he cited Eugene Braunwald's work with the device. In 1987, he teamed up with Reese Terry, an experienced medical device-company executive with training in electrical engineering. With money from venture capitalists and early investors, Zabara and Terry cofounded Cyberonics, with its headquarters in Houston, to produce the device for commercial sale.[118] In 1990, with an infusion of money from Pfizer, they started clinical trials.[119] Their sole product was the VNS device—and unless they could bring it to market, they would have no revenues, no profits, and no business. Getting approval from the FDA was essential.

Cyberonics set about earning that approval by providing the FDA with data from a clinical trial, code-named E03, which followed 114 patients with epilepsy for fourteen weeks. Half of them received low-level electrical stimulation of the vagus nerve (designated as the "sham," or control, arm), and half received high-level stimulation (presumed to be therapeutic).[120] Bad news followed: in 1994, after reviewing the data, the FDA denied approval of the VNS device to treat epilepsy, saying that the study provided insufficient proof of benefit. If Cyberonics wanted to win approval, the company would need more test subjects and would need to study them for a longer period of time.

The FDA decision was devastating. Cyberonics was running out of money and had already cut staff. The FDA's refusal to approve the device looked like it would spell death for the company. The CEO at the time, Allen Hill, resigned.

Stepping into the breach was Skip Cummins, a flamboyant venture capitalist who helped fund the start-up of Cyberonics in 1987 and had joined the board in 1988. Like everyone associated with the company, he knew that if they didn't win approval for the VNS device, the company would be dead in the water—in Cummins's words, Cyberonics would be "essentially a failed technology and [a failed] company." He describes the situation at the time of Hill's resignation:[121]

[Hill] lost confidence that we would ever get approval...he resigned...we had no CEO. At the time we were running out of money. Morale was terrible. Nobody believed in the science. Nobody wanted to invest in the company; the stock was basically pink sheets. The board was looking for anyone who would put their hand up [to replace Hill]...I figured what the heck, this thing works!

So Cummins threw his hat in the ring and was appointed CEO in 1995. He was ready to lead the charge on behalf of the upstart company: no one could bum-rush opponents better—or be more persuasive. An imposing six-foot-two-inch former college linebacker, Cummins, with his shaved head and nonstop intensity, has been described as a bully who uses his appearance and demeanor to intimidate. Even the notoriously abrasive hedge fund manager and television host Jim Cramer called Cummins the "most combative, most antagonistic CEO in America."[122] Antagonistic or not, he proved capable of crushing any opposition to the VNS device, whether scientific or regulatory.

This kind of industry aggressiveness with FDA staff was becoming the new normal. The rise of the biotech and medical device industries in the late 1970s unleashed a stampede of companies that sold just one or two products. Large pharmaceuticals companies with multiple products can generally afford a "miss" or a withdrawn drug. But the new biotech and device companies are often one-trick ponies that can't afford a loss: they are lean and hungry, and they market their sole prized products with a do-or-die mentality.

Cummins was unusually well suited for the role of CEO. He later observed, "When you're trying to commercialize a pioneering science that nobody believes in, that's not for a shrinking violet or the faint of heart."[121] Cummins went into discussions with the FDA in full battle gear, ready to take on what he says was an unreasonable demand by the agency. He relates the FDA's position on the first-ever medical device to treat epilepsy by stimulating the vagus nerve:

> FDA's biggest issue was: we don't really have a precedent for how we should approve or not approve a device for the treatment of epilepsy. We only have drugs that do that. We are going to hold you to a drug standard, which [requires] huge double-blind randomized controlled trials.[121]

Cummins was incensed. The FDA's standards for approval of medical devices are generally far lower than they are for drugs.[123] For the vast majority of implantable devices, the FDA doesn't require that clinical outcomes be tested; device manufacturers don't have to prove that their products improve clinical outcomes or make patients live longer. Instead, as one expert commented, the only thing manufacturers have to prove is that a device does what they say it will do—that a cardiac pacemaker fires electrical impulses at regular intervals, that a cardiac stent will increase blood flow through a previously blocked artery, or that an artificial hip actually bends and rotates as a hip should. Those questions are relevant and important. But they don't address the questions people care most about: Is this device safe, and will it help me live longer or feel better?

Furthermore, while the FDA doesn't require clinical data for most high-risk implanted devices, even the few devices that have undergone testing generally don't measure patient-oriented, clinically important outcomes, such as overall deaths. Instead, 88 percent tracked surrogate markers, such as laboratory tests and symptoms. But surrogate markers have frequently failed—and failed badly.

Consider coronary angiograms, the surrogate marker widely used to test the benefit of cardiac stents (stents are small metal tubes placed in coronary arteries to hold open arteries that are damaged or blocked by plaque). Angiograms are videos of the heart taken as dye is shot into the newly opened arteries, which often show blood squirting though previously blocked arteries where there had been little or no flow before. But as dramatic as such surrogate-marker evidence on an angiogram may appear, it isn't evidence that the patient will actually *do* any better clinically, that he or she will be any less likely to have a heart attack and die.

But because it seems perfectly logical that, if a coronary artery is blocked by plaque, and it is opened up with a stent, it would be a good thing, doctors—using this surrogate evidence—began implanting stents in millions of patients during percutaneous coronary angioplasty (PCI). The procedure seemed to work brilliantly.

It took years, and plenty of scientific argument, before a comprehensive study was performed to examine clinically important outcomes, such as future heart attacks and deaths. The results were disturbing: for patients undergoing PCI during elective surgery (as opposed to emergency surgery during an evolving heart attack), the procedure failed to prevent future heart attacks and deaths any better than simply treating patients nonsurgically, with medicines.[124] Disturbingly, a survey of cardiologists and patients with angina, or heart pain, found that two-thirds of the cardiologists acknowledged that the procedure would *not* prevent future heart attacks—yet 88 percent of patients believed it would protect them from heart attacks and death.[125, 126]

Although the procedure was reported to at least reduce symptoms, Bernard Lown, a now-retired Harvard cardiologist, said, "Optimizing medicine and life style achieves the same benefit as stenting at a far lower cost." But, he adds, "Stenting is a lucrative business." Dr. Rita Redberg, a cardiologist at the University of California at San Francisco and editor of *JAMA Internal Medicine*, said, "Many stents are placed in patients without symptoms or who have not been tried on medical therapy and thus are unnecessary," and, worse, "It is not clear that they actually reduce symptoms."[127–130] Citing the major study that compared PCI to treatment with medicines only, Redberg said that the small benefit in terms of chest-pain symptoms was gone after a few years[131, 132] and that percutaneous coronary interventions have never been tested in a blinded trial, so it is not possible to know if even the temporary benefit of pain relief is simply attributable to the placebo effect of the procedure. Compared to nonsurgical therapy, Redberg said, percutaneous coronary interventions "expose individuals to the harms of an invasive procedure with radiation, which increase[s] cancer risk, and [a] contrast agent, which poses threats to kidney function."

Vikas Saini, a cardiologist and president of the Lown Institute, says that researchers with the American College of Cardiology found that only half the patients who underwent stenting were deemed "appropriate," and while many of the other half were said to be of "uncertain appropriateness," financial and cultural incentives "completely align for almost all of them to get stented with no real incentives not to do it."

Just as stents were approved based on a surrogate marker of vessel openness on angiography, so Cyberonics sought approval of the VNS device on the basis of a reduction in seizures—also a surrogate marker. FDA reviewer Steven Piantadosi, professor of oncology and biostatistics and a clinical-trial methodologist at Johns Hopkins, commented on the unreliability of using a surrogate marker as a measure of success, especially in light of what he called the "high number of deaths" (seventeen of first one thousand) among VNS patients.[133] This was critically important, because Cyberonics emphasized the problem of deaths from epilepsy, with the implicit suggestion that the VNS device might reduce that risk by reducing seizures. In the official transcript of the FDA approval hearings, Piantadosi observes:

[O]ne of the things that's concerning me is that the endpoint being measured in all of these studies is, in some sense, a surrogate: counting the number of seizures. I realize that to the patient and to others, it is a very important endpoint, but it may not be as definitive as some other things that we could measure. There are numerous examples in the methodologic literature about the weaknesses of accepting clinical trial data based on surrogate outcomes...I would point to, as a recent and a very dramatic example, the cardiac arrhythmia suppression trial, in which the study was designed and the endpoint was selected on the basis of looking at arrhythmias and suppressing them with a drug.

And the studies originally seemed to show that the drug was effective in suppressing arrhythmias. The problem was that it was so good in suppressing arrhythmias that it was killing people, and the mechanism was not understood until much later and wasn't even believed until the results of the randomized trial.

So, I am very nervous when I see high mortality rates associated with a supposed benefit, even though we don't have a way biologically right now to connect the two. So, that is why I have harped on this this morning and why I am still very nervous with this high death rate....

The comparison of the VNS device in the treatment of seizures with anti-arrhythmic drugs in the treatment of abnormal heart rhythms is apt: both seizures and certain heart-rhythm disturbances are associated with an increased risk of death. Yet the CAST (Cardiac Arrhythmia Suppression Trial) showed that correcting heart-rhythm disturbances with certain drugs actually *increased* the risk of harm and death.[3] Could the same true for the VNS device? Only a study examining overall deaths could provide the answer. But that was another weak link in the way the VNS studies were designed: the device was never directly tested against a group of patients treated with medicines. Instead the studies measured only two different levels of electrical shocks, and one was likely to do better than the other by sheer chance. If the high-stimulation group did better, then it was a winner. If the low-stimulation group did better, the company could claim that the higher dose was just too high.

It's not even clear that individuals who did experience fewer seizures had the VNS device to thank. There are several reasons why patients enrolled in clinical trials tend to improve over their baselines. One is that during a trial they generally receive intensive care and oversight that's not part of "usual and customary" care. Another reason is "regression to the mean," which occurs in patients with chronic conditions that wax and wane (recall that Fegan's seizures varied enormously from month to month). Because patients tend to improve after periods of doing poorly, and because patients tend to enroll in clinical trials only when they are doing poorly (rather than when they are doing well), they are likely to improve simply because of the passage of time—in other words, they "regress to the mean," or average severity, of their condition. Then there's the placebo effect, which can also cause a patient to improve over baseline. One simple fact remains: what can't be determined from the Cyberonics studies is whether patients implanted with a VNS device will do any better (or worse) than they would if they were treated with medicines.

Although the FDA had set a low bar for Cyberonics by allowing seizure counts to serve as a metric of success without requiring patient-oriented clinical outcomes, CEO Skip Cummins was nonetheless seething.[121] He knew every detail of the FDA approval requirements, and he knew that plenty of implantable devices had gotten passes without having to conduct a single randomized trial, much less two. And he was worried that the cash-strapped Cyberonics would be unable to find funders to pay for a second study. The company was at its lowest point.

Despite seemingly insurmountable obstacles, Cummins charged ahead. He managed to persuade St. Jude Medical to invest $12 million in the company with an option to buy.[134] Cummins put the cash infusion from St. Jude to work in a second trial, dubbed E05, and the company included the results of E05 in a new submission packet to the FDA.

The E05 results, however, were far from impressive.[135] In fact, St. Jude Medical, which had made an offer of $72 million for the company, decided to withdraw the offer after the new results were revealed.

The E05 study divided 199 individuals with epilepsy into two groups and followed them for one year. As in the earlier study, E03, one group received "low stimulation," and the other group received "high stimulation." The high-stimulation group had an average 28 percent reduction in seizures compared to the low stimulation group, which experienced a 15 percent reduction. The difference didn't reach statistical significance, according to Piantadosi.[133] Yet somehow Cummins managed to persuade the FDA to approve the device. He returned triumphant from the 1997 meeting with the agency: the FDA had granted Cyberonics approval to market the VNS device for individuals with treatment-resistant epilepsy.

There was just one small glitch: the approval was given conditionally because of concerns about the high number of deaths, as noted by Piantadosi. Under conditional approval, the FDA can order a device off the market if the manufacturer fails to provide postapproval studies showing it to be safe. In other words, despite concerns that the device could be killing people, the company was able to sell it and attempt to prove its safety *after* it was on the market.

But that was a tiny bump in the road for Cyberonics. It won the approval it had been seeking, and it was now free to market the VNS device to doctors and the public at large. And since the FDA didn't require that the company disclose to doctors or patients that the device was effectively on probation because of concerns about high death rates, the public remained in the dark. Only the company and a handful of people at the FDA would know.

The 1997 triumph for Cyberonics in no small part due to the research Dr. Eugene Braunwald had done more than thirty years before, as the first expert to use vagus nerve stimulation to treat a medical condition. As I noted, Braunwald's pioneering work on the VNS was cited in numerous patent applications filed by Cyberonics. Unfortunately, the two deaths among just four patients that Braunwald had witnessed, along with his initial cautionary remarks, appear to have been forgotten by the time the FDA gave its blessing to Cyberonics.

Skip Cummins was thrilled. He later told *Forbes* reporter Robert Langreth that the VNS device is "a gigantic opportunity. We are talking about some of the largest medical markets in the world." He predicted, "Brain stimulation will be to the next 10 years what cardiac pacemakers were to the last 40."[117]

Cyberonics played up the comparison of the VNS device to a cardiac pacemaker. It was a useful marketing ploy: it evoked the image of a remarkably successful device. But the comparison is misleading. The cells of the heart react to the electrical stimuli of a pacemaker by contracting. It's a simple cause-and-effect response. The brain, on the other hand, is an exquisitely complex organ with myriad feedback loops. Twelve cranial nerves, of which the vagus nerve is one, transmit impulses to and from the brain. Each nerve interconnects with, responds to, and can affect countless other nerve cells that allow us to see, feel, touch, hear, and think. The crude application of an electrical impulse to a large nerve with multiple important functions—from regulating digestion and heart rate to providing feedback to the brain from virtually every major organ in the body—and expecting to reliably achieve a specified desirable outcome is not quite the same as applying an electrical impulse to heart cells that have a single simple function: to contract.

But none of that mattered to Cyberonics, which began to market its device directly to patients as well as doctors. While the company posted wildly positive testimonials on its website, there were no cautions in the promotional literature or videos about the seventeen deaths among the first one thousand patients implanted. Nor was there mention that the FDA had awarded only conditional approval of the device because of concerns about the high number of deaths, meaning that patients undergoing implantation were essentially guinea pigs in the quest to determine whether the device would be more likely to help them or kill them.

Between 1997 and mid-2005, sales of the VNS device were limited to the approximately thirty thousand individuals in the US with treatment-resistant partial epilepsy—a small subset of the estimated 2.4 million Americans with active epilepsy. Cyberonics needed to expand its market. Cummins was ready. The company had been taking out multiple patents on the VNS device, claiming that it could treat an array of medical problems, and the next condition the company wanted to tackle was depression.

Cyberonics said some epileptic patients experienced improvement in their moods after being implanted with the VNS device. This was potentially great business information. Depression is a huge healthcare crisis, affecting millions of Americans. If the VNS device could be sold as a treatment for depression, profits could dwarf those produced by the epilepsy market. The company launched a study to examine the role of VNS in depressed patients.

But the pivotal ten-week study of the VNS device in treating depression that Cyberonics submitted to the FDA was a bust: it showed no clinical benefit.[123, 136] To make matters worse for Cyberonics, Suzanne Parisian, a former chief medical device officer at the FDA, reacted to Cyberonics' failure to report sixty patient deaths during a single nine-month period, saying, "You have [sixty] people with epilepsy that had this implanted device [and] the FDA was never told that they died, and the company never did an investigation as to why they died, and the company's contending that the device is safe and effective. It's very unlikely that anybody will do any kind of an examination in these patients to find out why they're dying, and then you're asking them to expand the indication to depression patients."[137]

Despite the company's attempts to spin the depression study as positive, in 2004 the FDA issued a "non-approvable letter." The VNS could still be used to treat epilepsy—but not depression.

None of that was about to stop Skip Cummins. He knew just what to do—and he had the power to do it. He authorized $440,000 in lobbying expenditures in 2005 to persuade the FDA to reverse its position. The lobbying funds were significant for a small company, comprising more than it had spent during any other year (for example, in 2009, with no other applications pending, the company spent $8,000 on lobbying).[138]

Cummins personally lobbied the FDA, insisting that the agency would be guilty of abandoning depressed individuals to death by suicide if it failed to approve the VNS device for depression treatment. He pointed to one-year follow-up data that he said showed benefit—though experts with Public Citizen would later point out that the data came from a poorly designed, "non-randomized, unblinded, non-concurrent control group" and that a mandated FDA analysis found "no statistically significant benefit on any…outcome."[123, 136] Cummins took a new tack—he enlisted former Democratic House majority whip Tony Coelho to be on the board of Cyberonics.[139] Coelho's career was marred by scandal. He'd resigned from Congress in 1989 following reports that he participated in a sweetheart deal involving a "troubled S&L operator" and the purchase of a $100,000 junk bond, and in 1998 he was found to have vastly overcharged the US government to support a lavish lifestyle.[140] Nevertheless Coelho, who has epilepsy, proved to be a worthy ally to Cummins. After leaving Congress, he maintained extensive ties with top-level government officials and worked as Al Gore's campaign chairman. He crafted the Americans with Disabilities Act and later served as chairman of the board of directors of the Epilepsy Foundation. Given that Congress holds the purse strings, the FDA could hardly dismiss Coelho, whose influence continued to be felt in political circles.

By July of 2005, Cummins's strategy, with the help of Coelho, had paid off. The FDA approved the VNS device for "treatment-resistant depression."

But the approval by Daniel G. Schultz, then the director of the FDA's Center for Devices and Radiological Health, was awarded over the objections of nine FDA scientists who unanimously recommended against approval of the VNS device for the treatment of depression. It was the first time in the agency's history that an FDA director had overruled the unanimous recommendation of FDA scientists.[123, 136, 141] The resulting scandal, dubbed Devicegate, revealed that the agency had spied on the dissenting scientists, which led to a rancorous rebellion by nine of the scientists who filed a lawsuit against the agency. (We'll return to that story in a later chapter.)[142]

According to the Union of Concerned Scientists, "By overruling his scientific advisors, Dr. Schultz set in motion a potential windfall for Cyberonics."[141] The ruling led to a $2.3 million overnight gain, on paper, for Cummins. Together, Cummins and Coelho reaped $50 million by trading a money-losing stock: the company had raised $175 million from investors by 2006 while chalking up $186 million in losses.[139, 143]

Investors were positively giddy about the approval. The financial website Seeking Alpha urged readers to buy Cyberonics stock in a story headlined WHETHER YOU SUFFER FROM DEPRESSION OR NOT, DON'T MISS YOUR CHANCE TO PROFIT FROM IT. The article noted that the Centers for Disease Control and Prevention estimated that one in ten Americans suffers from depression and that *Healthline* estimated that the number of people being diagnosed was increasing by 20 percent per year. Since half of them wouldn't respond to the initial course of treatment, they predicted that about 5 percent of the US population (with a growth rate of 20 percent per year) would be candidates for the VNS device. Cyberonics estimated that some four million people in the US had treatment-resistant depression.

By then, Cyberonics was investigating some fifty-five conditions they thought the VNS device might be sold to treat, including anxiety, atrial fibrillation, autism, bulimia, burn-induced organ dysfunction, and drop attacks as well as fibromyalgia, heroin-seeking behavior, hiccups, multiple sclerosis, inflammation of the heart (myocarditis), obesity, rheumatoid arthritis, congestive heart failure, and ringing in the ears. The company had taken out patents for the device covering each of these indications.[77]

Cyberonics' proposition that such a bizarrely wide range of ills could be treated with one device is reminiscent of the claims made by hucksters of an earlier era. Consider the promoters of the Violetta machine, which in many ways was the forerunner of the VNS device. In the early 1900s, the manufacturers of the device claimed that electrical impulses generated by their machine and applied through the skin via various attachments could cure everything from back pain and carbuncles to a stuffy nose and foggy thinking, along with a host of other ills.

Among the scientific oddities that curator Denny Daniel displays in his traveling Museum of Interesting Things are several antique medical devices, some of which look like instruments of torture. At the 2017 BIOMEDevice convention and exposition in Boston, he held up one device that looked a bit like a necklace made of thin rope with a few decorative beads attached. The convention engineers and techies gathered around and giggled nervously as Daniel explained that the "necklace," which is attached to a "battery belt," is meant to be placed around a man's "special part." The intended result? To transform him into a more "manly man."

While there's nothing new about unscrupulous device makers hocking their wares, most of the quack devices of yore were used externally. Now modern technology allows these devices to be implanted *inside* us, sometimes making them far more effective—but also far more dangerous. For example, the conch shell hearing aid (a real conch shell used to funnel sound into the external ear canal) has given way to cochlear implants, which can improve hearing much more than a conch shell but which also can cause rare cases of fluid around the brain and meningitis. Daniel says he believes that many of today's devices will end up in a museum display much like his— for people to laugh and shake their heads at.

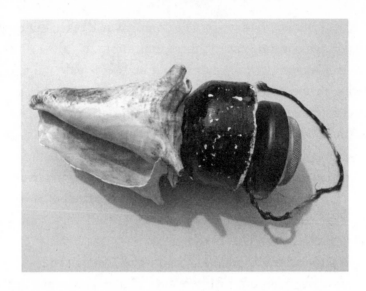

Early hearing aid: Conch Shell Ear Trumpet, widely used until the early 1900s, replaced by external hearing aids and cochlear implants.
(Image courtesy of Denny Daniel, Director, Museum of Interesting Things, New York City)

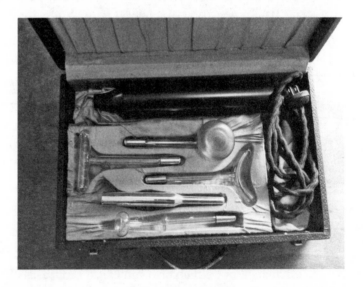

This Violetta machine (circa 1920) applied "violet rays" of low current to various parts of the body to treat "brain fog," stuffy nose, and impotence. Now implanted electrical devices are used for pain, Parkinson's, seizures, depression, and more. (Public domain)

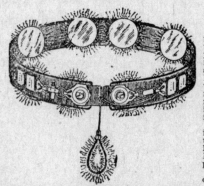
Dr. Sanden's electric belt (circa 1892) applied electricity to a man's "special part" to restore "life force" for a manly man. It was also said to treat kidney disease, nervous problems, backaches, rheumatism, congestion, and weakness. (Image courtesy of the Library of Congress)

From a business perspective, by 2005 Cyberonics could be viewed as a model of success in the world of the medical-industrial complex. It had used the pioneering work of a brilliant medical researcher, Eugene Braunwald, as the basis for building a burgeoning corporate empire. Unfortunately, the company's climb to success had required it to ignore some of the hints of danger in Braunwald's own study, to rely on research tests that provided only modest to nonexistent support for its claims of clinical benefit, and to use political influence to strong-arm a government regulatory agency into granting it approval over the objections of its own scientists.

Over time, these questionable tactics would come back to haunt Cyberonics. But in the short term, individual patients like Dennis Fegan, who put their lives in the company's hands, would pay a serious price.

Chapter Five

ADVERSE EVENTS

It wasn't long after Dennis Fegan was discharged from the hospital in 2006 that he discovered a website devoted to people who had been implanted with a VNS device. The website, which hosts a message board run by a woman named Donna Baum, would have an enormous impact on Fegan's future.

A friendly, round-faced woman with long dark hair, Baum recalls the intense anxiety she felt after her first seizure, which she had in 2001, at the age of forty-seven. Wanting information as well as the company of other people with her condition, she sought out an epilepsy support group. She found a local one led by an enthusiastic woman with epilepsy who told the participants she had had a device called a vagus nerve stimulator implanted in her chest to control her seizures. "She was so skinny," Baum recalls, "you could see [the VNS device] poking right out on her chest. She said it was the most wonderful thing."

Baum was eager to get help. Her seizure meds left her feeling groggy and confused. The suggestion that she might be able to use a device rather than drugs to control her seizures was a welcome prospect. So she, along with the rest of the group, was happy when the woman suggested bringing a Cyberonics representative to a meeting. They were even more delighted when they learned that the company would sponsor a free lunch presentation at a nearby hotel. When group members arrived, Cyberonics had placed a "gift bag" containing a promotional video and pamphlets on each person's chair. It was one of many such "seminars" held across the country at which people with seizures were told about the benefits of having a VNS device.

Afterward, Baum says the company began a lengthy period of "courting" her. "Cyberonics started taking interest in me from that very first meeting," she said, and she wasn't the only member of the support group the company pursued. In the months that followed, Cyberonics representatives, she said, would "take us out to lunch, call every week, and ask how we were doing." Baum was grateful for the attention. Fearful of having a seizure in public, she was hesitant to go out and mostly remained at home. The friendship of the Cyberonics representatives filled the void. They seemed to care about her. They listened to her with interest. And the free lunches were nice. "It wasn't just McDonald's, you know. They took us to Denny's."

She was especially excited to discover that Cyberonics sponsored a message board for patients on its website, a welcoming place for anyone with epilepsy, whether he or she had a device implanted or not. Here Baum found the community she had been seeking. People could discuss anything on the message board: the ins and outs of living with epilepsy, the mind-numbing drugs, the surgical options (including VNS), even personal problems. They cheered each other on, asked after each other, commiserated when things didn't go well; they understood each other. Baum says the support members gave each other "was incredible."

But not long after the message board was launched, disturbing posts began to appear.

As more people were implanted with the device, more complaints of unexplained symptoms surfaced. The message board began to resemble a complaint board, and anger mounted as the company failed to respond to questions. Were participants' symptoms caused by the VNS device?

Cyberonics staff, previously solicitous, suddenly turned cold. They no longer responded with pleasantries. Nor were they inviting Baum out for lunch anymore. Then, without fanfare, Cyberonics simply pulled the plug on the message board and shut it down. Adam Feuerstein, a biotech analyst writing for TheStreet.com, said the abrupt action followed mounting complaints by patients who posted comments "critical of the company and its device." One patient who posted critical comments, Elisa Driesen, told Feuerstein that the VNS "did nothing" to stop her seizures. She said the side effects of "constant pain, numbness, and breathing problems" were unbearable, adding, "My mission was to educate people...I wanted people to know what I was experiencing with the VNS. Now that the message board is gone, my greatest fear is that people won't be educated now."

Outraged that the company shut down the message board, Baum decided to take action. On February 18, 2004, one week after Cyberonics closed its message board, she opened a publicly accessible "VNS Message Board." Anyone who entered "VNS" or "vagus nerve stimulator" and "support group" into Google could find it.[144] So of course Dennis Fegan did, and his spirits lifted. Baum's message board didn't just connect him to others implanted with the VNS device, it was also a treasure trove of information.

Writing as "Birdbomb," Baum posted a link on the message board to the FDA's database of "adverse events," or possible side effects related to medical devices. The database, known as the Manufacturer and User Facility Device Experience (MAUDE), includes voluntary reports from hospitals, manufacturers, and others of side effects associated with medical devices as well as mandatory manufacturer reports of life-threatening events and deaths.

Fegan began the hunt for Cyberonics' report on his own experience. He recalled asking the Cyberonics representative, Steven Parnis, during their August 2006 encounter whether the company planned to file a report with the FDA about what had happened to him. Parnis did not give a straight answer to the question. Over the next few months, Fegan searched through thousands of reports of adverse events associated with the VNS device, and still no report from Cyberonics on his own incident appeared. Now Fegan understood why Parnis had been so noncommittal: it appeared that he may not have intended to file a report.

Parnis had also told Fegan and Bahamon that the company hadn't seen other cases like his. But late one night, sitting in his bedroom-cum-office, with the only light coming from his computer screen, Fegan came across a case report of a patient admitted to a hospital with an abrupt increase in seizures. The report said the patient was found to have "severe asystolia" coincident with vagus nerve stimulation.[145] By then, Fegan knew the words *asystole* and *asystolia* all too well. He could feel his pulse quicken. There it was—the very thing Cyberonics claimed hadn't happened to anyone else: a patient's heart had repeatedly stopped, and then, when the device was disabled, his normal heart rhythm was restored. Later, Cyberonics would claim that they had no reports of patients dying from asystole caused by the VNS device.[146] They conceded that they had four cases of asystole on file, but they said all of them occurred only during surgery and that all four patients recovered and did well.

Fegan wasn't convinced. He continued to dig into the MAUDE database and found a number of cases in which patients developed drop seizures, yet they would have other symptoms or signs not typical of drop seizures, such as losing consciousness and turning blue. His own episodes had been mistaken for drop seizures, though he was in fact losing consciousness because prolonged asystole was causing him to pass out.

A January 2004 report Fegan found on MAUDE read:

[Patient] originally received the VNS system so that he could reduce the medications he was taking. The VNS did not appear to help, and the patient began to have recurrent and more frequent events. The patient reported that 80 percent of the seizures are without warning...and has difficulty breathing...His lips will turn blue and he will fall from standing. [The patient was admitted to the hospital, where the following was observed:] He went from his prior sinus [normal] rate to a progressive bradycardia [slowing of the heart rate], culminating in a 15-second pause [asystole]... There was concern that the VNS system may have contributed to the event, therefore the VNS device was deactivated.

Here was another case similar to Fegan's and an important clue to the real diagnosis of asystole: the "seizures" stopped as soon as the VNS was turned off. Nonetheless, Cyberonics concluded that it was "exceedingly unlikely that the VNS device contributed to the episode of asystole." Another case report, dated January 1, 1999, described a patient who developed drop seizures after being implanted with the VNS. Once again, the device was turned off and the "seizures" stopped.

And there were more such cases. Many more.

The trail of clues that the device was indeed causing asystole was there for anybody to see in the MAUDE reports. Over time, Fegan became increasingly savvy about the FDA's MAUDE database. He soon learned how to sort "adverse events" according to the type of event. When he filtered the results for deaths, he was stunned by what he got back. There were hundreds of deaths associated with the VNS device. And many cases were similar to his experience.

By 2010, Fegan had plowed through approximately eight hundred VNS-related death reports on MAUDE. Because only fifty thousand or so patients had been implanted worldwide at the time, and because the device had only been on the market for eight years, the number of deaths was disturbing, especially since the average age of people implanted with the device during clinical trials was thirty-three. But despite hundreds of reports of death that contained very little information that could shed light on the cause, the company never attributed a single death to its device. In almost every instance, Cyberonics blamed sudden unexpected death in epilepsy (SUDEP) and concluded each report with the same sentence: "There is no evidence at this time that the [VNS] caused or contributed to the reported event."

But Fegan wondered, how could they know that?

For example, report 1246223:

Patient was found unresponsive and later passed away. Per reporter, patient had a lot of neurological problems, but was doing well with VNS with respect to seizures. An autopsy was performed and the autopsy report was obtained by the manufacturer. X-rays were taken and no anomalies were noted. The autopsy report noted the patient died of natural causes ascribed to a seizure disorder due to cerebral palsy. Due to the autopsy being an external examination versus complete autopsy and the circumstances surrounding the patient death, the manufacturer has classified this death as a probable SUDEP event.

No other information was provided. Fegan was baffled—an "autopsy" that consisted of an "external examination" and X-rays?

They looked at someone's dead body externally and decided the patient died of SUDEP? When I later asked Marcia Angell, a pathologist and former editor in chief of the *New England Journal of Medicine,* to comment on this report, she said wryly that she would love to have been able to conduct an autopsy by just looking at a dead body. "It would have made my work so much easier."

Neither sex nor age is indicated on MAUDE reports, but if report 1246223 was accurate, and the patient was "doing well with VNS," as stated, did that mean the patient didn't have a seizure—the very thing most associated with SUDEP? And if the patient didn't have a seizure,* how could anyone conclude that the death was "probable SUDEP"? Wasn't it equally plausible that the sudden and unexpected death was the fault of the VNS device?

Other deaths that Fegan found on MAUDE were equally concerning. For example:

[Patient] was under 24-hour video monitoring...died in 2009, due to [unknown] reasons...It is currently believed he died of a "terminal seizure," but the video...did not record a seizure.

And this:

Patient was found dead in their bed by caregiver. Cause of death is unknown...Manufacturer has determined that SUDEP is probable. The reporter has stated the [VNS device] was unrelated to the death....patient was walking into a room and simply dropped dead. Treating neurologist indicted that the death may be cardiac-related.

---

* SUDEP *can* occur in the absence of a seizure, but most often it is associated with a grand mal seizure.

As in so many other cases, Cyberonics reached its standard conclusion, stating, "There is no evidence at this time that the [VNS device] caused or contributed to the reported event."

Some reports consist of just a single sentence—"Patient found dead in bed" (or "in bathtub" or "on floor")—followed by the claim that the death was attributable to "probable SUDEP," which in turn would be followed by Cyberonics' standard conclusion that there was no evidence that the device "caused or contributed to" the patient's demise.

Fegan knew that if his parents hadn't shown up on that morning of July 2, 2006, and if he had died at home, there would be no EKG evidence to tell the real story, no observation by three doctors who all saw the same thing. "If I had died that day," he says, "they'd say I died of SUDEP." And Cyberonics would have reached the same conclusion as it did for everyone else: the VNS device never killed anyone.

There was an odd contradiction in the way Cyberonics interpreted bad versus good outcomes that may have contributed to underreporting of complications. When a patient developed problems months or years after implantation, Cyberonics would suggest that the VNS device was an unlikely cause, since the patient had, according to Cyberonics, "tolerated the VNS well" until that time. On the other hand, if a patient experienced a reduction in seizures months or even years after implantation, the company would attribute the reduction to the therapeutic effect of the device. Just why an electrical impulse, with its instantaneous effects, should fail to do the job for a year or longer is never explained. In the world of Cyberonics, delayed benefits could occur, but delayed harm could not.

In 2005, a year before Fegan had been hospitalized with asystole, he told his neurologist that the device wasn't helping him and asked to have it removed. According to Fegan, Bahamon encouraged him to hang on, saying it could take years for some patients to achieve benefit (Fegan had already had it in for more than four years at the time). The following year he was taken to the hospital with asystole. After that he wasn't about to fool around—he insisted on having it removed.

Bahamon referred him to a surgeon. But the surgeon told Fegan he wouldn't attempt to remove the wire leads from his vagus nerve. That was too risky. The surgeon explained that the leads often trigger inflammation and fibrosis (or scarring) that can progress for years after implantation. It was also possible that, with movement of the neck, the irritant effects of the leads pulling on the vagus could cause progressive enmeshment of the nerve in scar tissue and cause nerve dysfunction. He could take out the generator under his collarbone, but he'd leave the wires in place.

Fegan's case was not unusual. Some surgeons decline to remove the wire leads after disastrous experiences with previous patients—either their own or their colleagues'.

Fegan continued to explore the FDA's website. Eventually he came across a warning letter from the FDA to Cyberonics about the sixty unreported deaths. The letter, dated March 23, 2001, was addressed to then president and CEO Skip Cummins, and it summarized the findings of a site visit to Cyberonics headquarters in Houston that was conducted from January to early February of 2001. During the visit, the FDA uncovered files on sixty deaths that Cyberonics failed to report. And the agency determined that the VNS device "may have caused or contributed" to the deaths. The FDA reviewer found many other unreported instances of serious infections and adverse events.

Within weeks of the FDA's site visit, the company came up with records of twenty-three additional deaths, bringing the total number of previously unreported deaths to eighty-three. This was in early 2001, not long after mid-July of 1997, when the FDA first approved the VNS device to treat epilepsy. Eighty-three unreported deaths had to comprise a substantial portion of all deaths among patients with a VNS device at the time. It wouldn't be the last time the company would fail to report deaths and injuries among patients using the VNS device.

★ ★ ★

Most healthcare consumers assume that their physicians are so knowledgeable, caring, and dedicated that they would never recommend a course of treatment that could be risky or unlikely to provide significant benefit to them—and of course in some cases this assumption is perfectly valid. But in a world where new drugs, therapies, and devices are continually being devised and marketed—often by companies with aggressive growth ambitions—it's not always possible for physicians to be experts about every new product or service that becomes available.

Under the circumstances, ordinary citizens and some healthcare professionals might assume that government agencies such as the FDA serve as a protective shield, scrutinizing and evaluating new treatments before they go to market and permitting only those backed by solid scientific evidence to be sold.

This would be a wonderful thing if it were true. But in the real world, the medical research establishment and government regulatory agencies play this protective role only to a very limited extent.

Despite the aura of science that surrounds modern medicine, its practice has traditionally had only a modest relationship to the most rigorous, evidence-based scientific disciplines, such as chemistry and physics. Medicine is orders of magnitude more complex in many ways than chemistry or physics. Give a drug to—or implant a device in—a human being, and numerous physiochemical, neurological, and endocrine effects are triggered, which in turn set off feedback loops as the body attempts to regain homeostasis, the state of equilibrium or balance necessary for normal functioning. And then there are human feelings and perceptions and environmental input, all of which means that, unlike a chemistry experiment, in which combining the right chemicals in the right manner will reliably produce the same desired result every time, a medical experiment in which you combine a drug or medical device with a human being might have any number of outcomes.

But that doesn't mean that science can or should be ignored when drugs and devices are developed. Medicine is all based on likelihoods: Is a person more likely to die if he or she has a pacemaker implanted? Will a person with epilepsy be more—or less—likely to die suddenly after implantation with a VNS device? Scientific evidence can help to answer such questions when well-designed studies are implemented. Yet history shows that hard evidence has played, and continues to play, only a modest role in the process by which medical treatments become widely popular. In fact, the search for truth based on experiment, or clinical trials, has shown up like the light of a firefly throughout medical history—flashing on for a moment, then going dark for long periods.

During the early modern period—the eighteenth and nineteenth centuries—experienced doctors simply taught younger doctors what they believed to be true from their own experience. In general, there was very little, if any, science involved in their practices. In this way, opinion and anecdote guided the choices doctors made about what tests and surgeries to perform and what drugs to administer. But experience can be misleading, paving the way for false conclusions and conflicting claims.

During this same period, the role of government in testing and regulating medical treatments was minimal. The Division of Chemistry, later the Bureau of Chemistry, the forerunner of today's FDA, was focused simply on ensuring that drugs weren't adulterated or "misbranded," meaning that a product contained the actual ingredients stated on the label. In 1906, the passage of the Federal Food and Drugs Act gave the bureau its first modest regulatory responsibilities.[147] But it had no role in ensuring that products were either safe or effective. Indeed, the US Supreme Court ruled in 1911, in *United States v. Johnson,* that the 1906 act did not prohibit false therapeutic claims.

The mandate of the Food and Drug Administration (as it was named in 1930) did not include safety requirements until the passage of the 1938 Food, Drug, and Cosmetic Act, after a disaster with a drug known as Elixir Sulfanilamide, a preparation used to treat strep throat. The drug contained diethylene glycol, a substance related to antifreeze, which killed more than one hundred children and adults in 1937. The safety standards set by the FDA in 1938 were far from rigorous, however. Manufacturers could, and often did, submit statements of expert opinion rather than well-controlled experiments as evidence of safety.

This began to change with the thalidomide disaster of 1961. Thalidomide was widely prescribed in Europe at the time to treat nausea. Manufacturers gave samples of the drug to thousands of doctors in the US, who in turn gave them to their patients (the drug had not been approved by the FDA at the time). Women who were pregnant when they took the drug gave birth to babies with deformities known as phocomelia, in which the arms and legs fail to develop. Many were born with what looked like small flippers or webbed fingers growing out of their shoulders and hips.

The FDA determined that mothers had been given the drug without being informed that it was "experimental," because it hadn't been approved in the US. This led to the 1962 Kefauver-Harris Amendments to the Food, Drug, and Cosmetic Act, which required—for the first time—that drugs have to be "efficacious" in order to win FDA approval. As with safety requirements, however, the bar was not set very high.

The first truly scientific test of a proposed new drug, a randomized controlled trial of streptomycin in the treatment of pulmonary tuberculosis, was conducted in 1946. Randomization means that researchers assign volunteers to either an experimental treatment group or a control group through a process intended to ensure that both groups are likely to be the same in terms of disease severity, age, and other factors that could affect outcomes. Use of control groups means that researchers can observe whether the experimental treatment actually makes a difference.

Too often however, devices and drugs are tested with either no control group or against a "straw-man comparator," in which a new treatment is tested against an older treatment (i.e., a comparator drug) in which the comparator drug is given in a dose or manner—such as a very low dose—that is less likely to be effective, making the new treatment look superior. Joe Lex, an emergency physician, once described the problem of strawman comparators after he reviewed all studies of a class of non-narcotic painkillers. "Guess what?" Lex said. "Whoever sponsored the study always got a better result than [the competitor]. In forty-eight percent of trials, the reason for that was because the dose of the sponsored drug was appropriate, but the dose of the drug that it was being compared to was less than appropriate. The straw-man study."[148, 149] Richard Lehman, a renowned British physician, said, "Straw-man comparators are a breach of ethics. Or, to put it another way, standard practice."

Patients and doctors routinely overestimate the dangers of various diseases and underestimate the harmful effects of treatments, making it easier for manufacturers to promote their products even when those products are never tested against a control group.[150, 151] A cancer drug might be reported as having an excellent 75 percent survival rate (which generally means that five years after treatment, 75 percent of patients are still alive). But the question is, how many people would have died *without treatment?* Many of the most deadly pandemics in history have had mortality rates of 25 percent—meaning that 75 percent survive anyway. Proper control groups, composed of either untreated patients (if no effective treatment is available for comparison) or patients treated with a known cure or therapy, are critical to determining whether a drug is making a difference.

Cyberonics was right to include the "sham" low-stimulation group, which was intended to reduce the possibility of the placebo effect by keeping patients in the dark about which group they were in. But the failure to include a third group, treated with medicines only, leaves the most basic questions unanswered: Does the device improve outcomes, and is it safe when compared to optimal drug treatment? It would be many years before an answer to those questions would be published, and it would come from a surprising source. (More on that later.)

The failure to use control or comparison groups continues to be a problem. For example, in 2015, the Centers for Disease Control and Prevention launched a campaign urging the public to take the "lifesaving" flu drug oseltamivir (Tamiflu), which is manufactured by Roche.[152] However, years earlier the FDA had issued a warning to Roche that it could not claim the drug saves lives or reduces pneumonia from flu, because the studies they provided to the FDA failed to demonstrate these outcomes.[152] Subsequent high-quality independent analyses of both published and unpublished Tamiflu data have failed to find any lifesaving benefit to the drug.[153] Despite this, the CDC went ahead with its Tamiflu campaign—basing its claim on case reports and observational studies. But without a control group for comparison, it's impossible to say whether the drug has actually saved a single life.[153] Unbeknownst to doctors and the public, the highly visible CDC campaign promoting Tamiflu was quietly paid for by Roche, the manufacturer of Tamiflu.[152]

To this day, drug and device manufacturers commonly promote their wares using studies that are inherently biased. John P. A.

Ioannidis, professor of health research and policy at Stanford University School of Medicine, has studied the claims of medical researchers published in the most prestigious medical journals. He found that most published research findings are false or exaggerated and that many clinical trials fail to yield the same results when replicated.[154, 155]

With industry bias wielding increasing influence in the halls of academe, the hope of genuinely independent inquiry has gradually faded. Many practicing doctors now feel they don't know which research claims they can trust. In 2006, the *American Journal of Psychiatry* published an amusing take on the problem of research bias. The authors noted that when manufacturers compare their drugs in head-to-head clinical trials, virtually all drug makers claim their drug is superior to all other drugs in the same class. The article was playfully entitled "Why Olanzapine Beats Risperidone, Risperidone Beats Quetiapine, and Quetiapine Beats Olanzapine."[156] The result is what Shannon Brownlee, vice president of the Lown Institute, calls the Lake Wobegon effect: where all drugs are above average.

Few healthcare consumers realize what a limited role impartial research plays in shaping the medical treatments they receive. In a poll conducted by the Campaign for Effective Patient Care, a nonprofit advocacy group based in California, 65 percent of the eight hundred California voters surveyed said they thought that most or nearly all the healthcare they receive is based on scientific evidence.[157] The reality would probably shock them. A panel of experts convened in 2007 by the prestigious Institute of Medicine estimated that "well below half" of the procedures doctors perform and the decisions they make about devices, surgeries, drugs, and tests have been adequately investigated and shown to be effective. The rest are based on a combination of guesswork, theory, and tradition, along with a strong dose of marketing by drug and device companies. Distinguishing false from true medical claims is a serious challenge; that's why the way studies are designed and carried out is so important. As FDA historian Suzanne White Junod observes, "The function of the formal controlled clinical trial is to separate the relative handful of discoveries which prove to be true advances in therapy from a legion of false leads and unverifiable clinical impressions."[147] The reality of medical science is that the vast majority of highly touted, seemingly promising cures—whether they take the form of new drugs, new therapeutic regimens, new surgical techniques, or new medical devices—simply don't work.

This is not a message that the ambitious, profit-oriented corporate leaders of the medical-industrial complex are eager to embrace. And so it's no wonder they have used their power and influence to resist attempts by medical researchers and some government agencies to challenge their claims or insist on more reliable scientific evidence to ensure that their products are safe and effective before they are approved by the FDA.

The emergence of fast-growing, ambitious companies like Cyberonics in the 1970s, '80s, and '90s posed significant challenges for the US medical regulatory system. Agencies like the FDA are supposed to safeguard the health and safety of the public. Yet given the complexity, size, wealth, and power of today's medical-industrial complex, that's a nearly impossible task for an underfunded agency subject to control by politicians beholden to industry.

Theoretically, the system for ensuring the safety of drugs and devices after they are approved for sale is supposed to work this way: The FDA receives reports from doctors, manufacturers, and hospitals in its adverse-events database. If an unusually high number of problems is reported—"red flags," as the agency puts it—the FDA can request a scientific study to determine whether a drug or device is causing a problem. But as Dennis Fegan began to discover by studying the MAUDE database, the FDA's red-flag system is hamstrung by a series of problems.

First, as the FDA itself acknowledges, its assessment of medical device safety is hampered by manufacturers and hospitals that submit "incomplete, inaccurate, untimely, unverified, or biased data."[158] One problem is that reporting is voluntary. Although manufacturers and facilities (hospitals) are required to report serious adverse events, doctors and other healthcare providers are not required to do so. As Diana Zuckerman, president of the National Center for Health Research, in Washington, DC, points out, even when facilities learn of a device problem, they often fail to report it to the FDA—nor does the FDA enforce the reporting requirement.[159] The upshot is that underreporting is commonplace, and only a tiny fraction of adverse events and deaths related to medical devices is ever reported. Zuckerman adds that there are "huge disincentives" for doctors when it comes to reporting adverse events: reporting takes time, and doctors are time-pressured already, with just minutes to see each patient.[159]

Even more important, Zuckerman said, is that doctors worry about being sued, and "they know that they will be blamed for problems [with devices] as the manufacturers [virtually] always say a bad outcome was due to 'operator error' (meaning that a doctor or patient used the device in an unapproved manner)," thereby exculpating the manufacturer. This is dangerous territory not only for patients but also for doctors, who are often lured by manufacturers that encourage doctors to use devices in an off-label manner, because it increases market share. But when something goes wrong, the manufacturer will say it bears no responsibility because the doctor used the product in an unapproved manner. As a result, patients drop product-liability suits against manufacturers and instead charge the healthcare provider with malpractice.

The only incentive to report, said Zuckerman, "is caring about patient outcomes, but that incentive generally isn't enough to overcome the disincentives." Companies like Cyberonics, which are financially dependent on a single device, have every reason in the world to want to hide or obfuscate evidence that might suggest that the device is dangerous.

The FDA requires that if a death or serious injury "reasonably suggests" that a drug or device "may have caused or contributed" to death or injury, the manufacturer must report the event to the FDA. But if it's determined that serious harm was not the fault of a drug or device, the company doesn't have to report it.

So who decides whether a device "caused or contributed" to a serious complication or death? The FDA leaves that decision up to the manufacturer.[100]

Mark E. Bruley, vice president of accident and forensic investigation at ECRI, an independent nonprofit patient-safety organization based in Plymouth Meeting, Pennsylvania, says there is a reason to allow companies not to report all deaths: "Virtually every patient who dies in a hospital dies on a stretcher, but we don't want stretcher manufacturers to report every hospital death." Such reports, said Bruley, would have no patient safety or regulatory value.[160]

Although Bruley's point is well taken, leaving it up to a manufacturer to determine whether its product was the cause of a patient's death throws open the doors to powerful biases—biases made all the more evident by imagining how different the conclusion might be if the patient's doctor or family were to make the determination. Manufacturers have powerful incentives to reach conclusions that don't implicate their drugs or devices, and there is almost always a plausible alternative explanation for individual events.

Allowing manufacturers to be the "deciders" amounts to a virtual get-out-of-jail-free card for device makers—an escape hatch from responsibility that must be tremendously tempting for even well-intentioned company employees. Of course, the FDA can overrule an obviously bad decision by a manufacturer, but out of the hundreds of thousands of reports filed in the MAUDE database, only a relative handful are challenged by the agency. Yet it is a disinterested third party and independently conducted studies that are most needed in these instances.

In Dennis Fegan's case, Steve Parnis, the Cyberonics staffer present at Fegan's August 2006 visit with Bahamon, was tasked with ferreting out the "root cause" of Fegan's brush with death.[161] Parnis was no ordinary Cyberonics employee with merely the usual incentive to protect his employer and his job. Unbeknownst to Fegan, between 2003 and 2005, the company had filed eight patents on the VNS device in Parnis's name, including one co-filed with Jacob Zabara, the original patent holder, in 2003.[162–169] This may have given Parnis, a senior manager with Cyberonics, an incentive to protect the reputation of the device and that of the company that manufactured and marketed it. Yet it was Parnis, a radiology technologist whose training consisted of a one-year program to become an invasive cardiovascular technologist,* who examined Fegan's EKGs and then wrote the official corporate report on the cause of Fegan's asystole.[161]

The fact that manufacturers can decide whether their own products do or do not contribute to an adverse event severely limits the value of the FDA's reporting requirement.

There are still other problems with the way the FDA tracks data about the safety of medical devices. For example, the agency does not collect data on the total number of devices (or drugs) on the market. This lack of a denominator makes statistics about the number of injuries all but useless. If there are fifty deaths among thirteen million users, that's very different from fifty deaths among two thousand users.

The FDA's failure to take full advantage of the potential power of

---

* Interventional cardiovascular specialists are trained to assist surgeons as they conduct cardiac catheterizations. Parnis declined to discuss his role in evaluating Fegan's asystole, and referred questions to Cyberonics.

the MAUDE database has become increasingly glaring in today's era of "big data." A fully functional, truly comprehensive MAUDE database could be a powerful tool for safeguarding patient health and ensuring the efficacy of drugs and devices. But it would take wide-ranging changes to the system.

Madris Tomes knows more than most experts about the short-comings of MAUDE. After graduating from American University with an MBA, she worked as a consultant with Booz Allen Hamilton, a management consulting company, and became adept at computer analytics—the craft of examining oceans of data to find patterns that mean something. Tomes went on to spend seventeen years in health information technology, mostly as a consultant to the Centers for Medicare and Medicaid Services and the FDA but also as an employee of the FDA itself.[170]

While working with the FDA's MAUDE database, she realized that researchers who relied on the agency's database would be misled if they didn't know how to mine the data as she did, since a portion of deaths was misfiled. Although the FDA was in the process of purchasing new software, when Tomes conducted an analysis using the new product, she says she found that it "will not perform the big data analytics that are vital to ensure patient safety."

Tomes decided to leave the agency to form her own company, Device Events, where she developed a program (at a price that she says was a mere fraction of the rumored $60 million the FDA paid for its program). The agency declined to review Tomes's software tool.

After she left her work with the FDA, she presented a demonstration of her database tool to Art Sedrakyan, a professor of healthcare policy and research and cardiothoracic surgery at Weill Cornell Medical College. He was having trouble tracking harmful consequences associated with Essure, an implanted medical device intended to provide permanent sterilization for women. The device, manufactured by Bayer, consists of two thin coiled wires about an inch long, which are inserted through the cervix and uterus into the fallopian tubes, where they cause a dense inflammatory reaction and scarring. The scarring in turn blocks eggs from descending into the uterus, where they could be fertilized. But the device can migrate and cause severe pain, bleeding, infections, and even perforation of internal organs, including the uterus and fallopian tubes.[171–174] Sedrakyan and his colleagues wanted to know how often these problems arose.

Tomes says Sedrakyan found "only a few hundred" adverse events related to Essure in the FDA's database. But, she says, "when I plugged [the word *Essure*] into my database, I got back over a thousand adverse events." As of July 2016, she said in a telephone call to me, the number stands at "well over twelve thousand adverse events."

Using Tomes's database, electronic health records, and claims data, Sedrakyan and his colleagues found that within a single year, one of every twenty-five women implanted with the Essure underwent surgery to have it removed, most often because of bleeding and pain, and they were ten times as likely to have to undergo reoperation as women who underwent a different sterilization procedure.[175]

The FDA awarded expedited approval to the device in July of 2002 based on the manufacturer's claim of a 99.8 percent success rate.[171] However, during the approval hearings, it was determined that the claim was based on the first year of use only: at two years of use, only 149 of 507 women in the study (a rate of 29 percent) were even evaluated, and there was no report on how effective it was among those women. At three years of use, only five of 507 women (a rate of 1 percent) had been evaluated.[176] The success claimed by Bayer was undermined by low follow-up rates and frequent complaints of miscarriages and unintended pregnancies.[176, 177]

The twenty thousand or so women complaining of pain, perforations, miscarriages, and the need to undergo surgeries and abortions caught the attention of activist Erin Brockovich. She took up their cause and joined them in demanding that that the FDA withdraw approval of the device. She deplored the FDA's inaction, saying that if "20,000 penises were falling off, the world would stop."[178]

When Tomes dug further into her database for fetal deaths related to Essure, only five deaths popped up in the MAUDE database using the "deaths" filter. But when she used her program, 303 deaths appeared—sixty times as many. She took her concerns to Congressperson Mike Fitzpatrick of Pennsylvania, who queried the FDA about her finding, and as a Fitzpatrick staffer put it, the agency confirmed that her finding was "spot on." In a letter to Fitzpatrick, the FDA acknowledged that it had 296 deaths on file, saying that the difference between 296 and 303 was simply "methodological."[179] Whether the correct number was 296 or 303, it was a far cry from the five deaths reviewers would see using the FDA's "deaths" filter.

Fitzpatrick sponsored a bill calling for the FDA to withdraw its approval for Essure, helping trigger an FDA hearing on the device. Although the agency ultimately declined to order the device removed from the market, it did order that a "black box" warning must be placed on the device label and that a checklist of cautions must be provided to patients before they undergo the procedure. However, severe underreporting of device complications continues to plague the FDA and its MAUDE database.

When problems with the FDA's database surfaced during public protests by women over safety issues related to Essure, a WNBC television reporter asked Tomes which device was the worst in terms of discrepancies in the MAUDE database. It didn't take long for her to come up with an answer: the vagus nerve stimulator. On August 3, 2016, Tomes conducted a side-by-side comparison between deaths associated with VNS device found in the MAUDE database and deaths found in the Device Events database. During 2015, there were only 206 deaths in the MAUDE database, while the Device Events database yielded 2,093 deaths. Since 1997, when the VNS device first came on the market, through June 30, 2016, the disparity was even worse: there were 2,006 death reports in the MAUDE database, while the Device Events database yielded 11,223 death reports. Making matters worse, the FDA has deleted from their online database all adverse events dating back ten years or more, while Tomes has twenty years of FDA data.

Of course no one knows how many of the deaths reported in the MAUDE database are actually deaths caused by the device. Many are likely to be unrelated. Nor do the additional deaths found in the Device Events database mean that each death was caused by the device. In many other cases, however, the device may well be the cause of death or serious harm.

The FDA acknowledges significant limitations of the MAUDE database. It acknowledges that it can't determine causality on the basis of individual reports, nor can it determine the true rate of harmful events caused by a particular device, because it doesn't track the number of devices in use. What the agency does say is that the database helps it to detect red flags—a sudden uptick in the overall number of adverse events or the occurrence of new or unexpected injuries could cause the agency to ask the manufacturer to conduct a safety study.

But as reports pile up in the MAUDE database, it's unclear if and when the agency is actually watching for red flags. A number of devices, including the VNS, have large numbers of deaths that failed to trigger action by the FDA.

The FDA responded to Tomes's findings by stating, "The [MAUDE] database and analysis tools allow the FDA to distinguish mentions of deaths...and those where the device caused or contributed to a death." Tomes said if that's true, the FDA is not making that clear by moving the misclassified deaths into the "deaths" category, as the case with Essure demonstrated.

Yet these discrepancies refer only to data already in the FDA's database. They pale in comparison to a far more significant problem acknowledged by the FDA itself as well as by the Government Accountability Office, which revealed in 1986 that hospitals report fewer than 1 percent of adverse device events to the FDA. According to the report, "the more serious the problem with a device, the less likely it was to be reported."[102] Put another way, 99 percent of device-related adverse events never make it into the FDA's database.

Sometime after 2010, the FDA removed that statistic—cited by former FDA commissioner David A. Kessler—from its website, but when questioned, the agency did not offer any newer statistic on underreporting.

Given the multiple uncertainties about the MAUDE database, the FDA's surveillance of negative outcomes appears to be as effective as using a Ouija board. And as we'll see, the problems with MAUDE are all too typical of the many shortcomings of the FDA. The sad truth is that guesswork, not science, is the main source for the agency's assurances of safety.

Chapter Six

NO SAFETY NET

BACK IN 2006, SHORTLY after Fegan's encounter with Steven Parnis of Cyberonics, his neurologist, Juan Bahamon, formally dropped Fegan from his patient roster. Fegan was unable to find another neurologist until 2008, two full years after his hospitalization. Eventually he found Dr. JoAnne Sullivan.* His family accompanied him to some of his visits, and both Fegan and his family took an enormous liking to her. Sullivan was compassionate. She explained things. She seemed to genuinely care about Fegan and showed concern when he told her about his terrible experience with the VNS device.

Fegan was still eager to obtain justice for his brush with death. But by 2008, he had begun to despair of getting help. He had contacted the FDA, state regulators, politicians, and the media and gotten nowhere. No longer embroiled in day-to-day skirmishes with various regulators and agencies, he settled into daily searches through the medical literature and the MAUDE database, scrutinizing new

---

* This is a pseudonym.

reports as they came in, hoping to find something, anything, that would turn things around.

His days took on a steady rhythm. He rarely went out, saying, "Something could happen and I wouldn't know it"—an oblique reference to having a seizure in public. His life as an outgoing, hail-fellow-well-met kind of guy who liked the beach, jogging, and square dancing was over. His world had contracted. On occasion, if a friend with a car came to visit, he might get a ride to the grocery store. But he would breathe a sigh of relief when he got home again and was alone, for it was only then that he felt comfortable.

It was during this slowed-down period, in May of 2008, when he pulled a letter from his mailbox and was surprised by the return address. The letter was from an unexpected source—the law firm of Winckler & Harvey, LLP, in Austin, Texas. He had contacted them more than a year earlier, along with "nearly a hundred" other law firms. None wanted to take his case. But now here was a response. Finally someone was following up. He found himself almost unwittingly giving in to hope. He knew better. He'd been disappointed so many times before. But still...he opened the letter. In amazement, he read that representatives from Cyberonics, who had previously disavowed any responsibility for Fegan's near-death experience, advised the law firm that they were "reconsidering their position on settlement."[180]

Fegan's hopes soared. A settlement! That was good. And while it wasn't as good as a trial, it was better than nothing.

A week or two later, Fegan received a call from one of the lawyers. He had no idea what to expect.

Fegan doesn't remember the exact amount of money the lawyer told him Cyberonics was offering. He does recall that it was less than $20,000. An amount that didn't even cover the hospital costs he and his insurance company paid.

Then, three weeks later, he pulled another letter from his

mailbox. He hadn't given the lawyers a definite answer about the offer. Maybe that was a good thing. Maybe the pathetic settlement offer by Cyberonics had persuaded the attorneys to take his case to court. He recalls, "I tore the letter open. I wanted my day in court. I was so anxious to move forward. Now maybe the FDA would have to listen."

But his excitement turned to disbelief as he read the letter, signed by attorney Jay Winckler: "I must inform you that you have no basis to file a lawsuit, and I therefore cannot take legal action on your behalf due to the recent U.S. Supreme Court ruling, In re: Riegel v. Medtronic, Inc., 552 U.S. 312 (2008), which bars claims against a manufacturer regarding the safety or effectiveness of a medical device."[181, 182]

Fegan had to read the sentence several times. The new ruling meant that no one could sue a manufacturer over a device if the device had been approved by the FDA. *Riegel v. Medtronic* meant it was all over. That was it. There would be no settlement. No suit. No nothing. Fegan's last avenue of redress had been shut down.

* * *

The Supreme Court ruling, based on a suit brought by Charles R. Riegel and his wife, Donna, against the medical device company Medtronic,[182] had been issued just months before the lawyers finally sent their letters to Fegan. Riegel had been undergoing angioplasty (a procedure to open a blocked coronary artery) with the Evergreen catheter, a device manufactured by Medtronic,[181] consisting of a catheter with a balloon on its leading edge. The catheter was threaded through an artery into the left side of Riegel's heart and from there into a blocked coronary artery. When the doctor inflated the balloon to open the artery, the balloon ruptured. Riegel went into complete heart block and lost consciousness. Placed on life support and rushed into emergency surgery to repair the damage, he was left with severe and permanent disabilities and died several years later, in 2004.

The Riegels contended that the catheter was defective and had caused grave harm. Their lawyers argued that this was a classic example of the kind of case for which a personal-injury lawsuit is the ideal—and often the only—remedy. They asserted in oral argument that "FDA regulation alone may not adequately protect consumer safety. Without the threat of lawsuits, manufacturers may hide information about device harms from the FDA during and after the [premarket approval (PMA)] process. Because the FDA does not conduct its own studies into device safety, the PMA process typically relies on those provided in the manufacturer's application, which may exclude those with unfavorable results."

For most of its history, the FDA itself had supported cases like the one brought by the Riegels. FDA administrators had long held that the right to sue was necessary to help compensate patients harmed by drugs and devices and potentially prevent future deaths and injuries and protect the public.[183] But by the time the Riegel case reached the Supreme Court, something had changed. Dan Troy, the general counsel for the FDA, had submitted an unprecedented friend-of-the-court brief in the Riegel case supporting the medical device industry's position, which advocated the so-called doctrine of preemption.[183] This doctrine would prohibit suits against makers of devices that have previously been approved by the FDA on the grounds that the agency's approval process makes any additional health or safety requirements unnecessary and, indeed, onerous and unfair. Since lawsuits in state courts (where personal-injury suits are filed) effectively threaten to establish requirements that are different from or additional to those of the FDA, Troy argued that such suits should be preempted.

That's exactly the logic that the Supreme Court relied upon in its

Riegel ruling. Justice Antonin Scalia, writing for the eight-to-one majority, said that states can't impose requirements that are different from or additional to those established by the FDA. He concluded that the twelve hundred hours spent by the FDA reviewing premarket applications for high-risk devices offer "reasonable assurance" that they are safe and effective.

Called the ten-thousand-pound gorilla of device rulings, *Riegel v. Medtronic* deprived many individuals such as Riegel (and Dennis Fegan) of redress.[184, 185] What's more, by preempting lawsuits that could bring safety problems to light, it deprived the general public of important information that could protect other healthcare consumers.

The ruling on preemption relies entirely on the FDA's device-approval process to ensure that devices are safe and effective. So let's examine the agency approval process—in particular what the FDA calls its "stringent" processes used for high-risk and implanted devices.

* * *

Medical devices didn't come under regulatory control by the FDA until 1976, when Congress passed the Medical Device Amendments (MDA) to the Food, Drug, and Cosmetic Act. The act followed on the heels of a scandal involving the Dalkon Shield, an intrauterine device designed to prevent pregnancy that was first marketed in 1971 as a safer alternative to birth control pills.[186] Just three years after the device went on the market, two and a half million women were implanted with the device. A design flaw allowed bacteria to enter the uterus, and thousands of women had to be hospitalized with serious infections. There were also a number of fatalities.[187, 188]

Because devices like tongue depressors and crutches don't need the same oversight as cardiac pacemakers, the FDA stratifies devices according to level of risk and need for clinical studies: low-risk (class I) devices include items such as scalpels and bandages; medium-risk (class II) devices include endoscopes and most total joint implants (such as most artificial hips and knees); high-risk (class III) devices include cardiac pacemakers, implanted defibrillators, deep-brain stimulators—and the VNS device.

Most class I and some class II devices are exempt from clearance or approval and can simply be registered with the FDA. For the remaining devices in classes I and II, the manufacturer simply has to notify the FDA of the product's class and its intent to market the device ninety days before distribution. The process, known as the 510(k) process, does not require clinical trials, and such devices are said to be cleared for market rather than approved.

Class III, or high-risk, devices are generally expected to undergo a premarket approval (PMA) process in which the manufacturer must provide "reasonable assurance" of safety and efficacy. However, one of the concessions won by the medical device industry was an allowance that all devices, including high-risk devices, on the market before 1976 could continue to be sold under the 510(k) provision. In addition, any new device that a manufacturer deems to be "substantially equivalent" to an existing device (known as a predicate device) could be eligible for clearance under the 510(k) provision. Even devices that are substantially equivalent to other devices cleared under the 510(k) process can be similarly cleared by the FDA, allowing potentially infinite iterations, a problem known as "predicate creep."[123] In this way, devices can change over time, the same way that a game of telephone can distort an original statement.

Addressing the 2009 annual meeting of the Medical Device Manufacturers Association, the director of the FDA's Center for Devices and Radiological Health, Daniel Schultz, acknowledged the problem with the 510(k) process, saying, "[There are situations] where we started with one device a long time ago and ended up some place very, very different. And it is really hard to explain that entire complicated path that got us from where we were in 1976 to 2009."[189]

The 1976 Medical Device Amendments were intended to ensure that high-risk devices would undergo scientifically valid clinical testing. Yet three decades later, only 16 percent (170 of 1,062) of the highest-risk devices approved by the FDA had gone through the PMA process. The rest had been either cleared without clinical testing through the 510(k) process (21 percent) or approved by supplemental filing (63 percent). Of the latter, only 0.3 percent were required to provide clinical data.[13, 14, 190] Supplemental applications are submitted by manufacturers to the FDA for changes to a device (such as new or upgraded models) that could affect effectiveness or safety—or when the manufacturer proposes a change in the label to include new diseases or conditions for which the device is intended.

Even when devices did undergo clinical testing, a 2009 study of seventy-eight applications for high-risk cardiovascular devices found that only 27 percent of studies (33 of 123) were randomized, only 14 percent were blinded, 88 percent of the primary end points were surrogate markers, roughly half of the studies had no control group, and nearly a third of those that did were retrospective—a form of review that is generally not as scientifically sound as a randomized controlled trial.[15]

A study published in the *JAMA*, the *Journal of the American Medical Association*, found that from 2008 through 2012, the FDA cleared for market approximately four hundred implanted medical devices considered of moderate to high risk—without requiring clinical testing.[191] This means that manufacturers have been able to sell everything from filters inserted into the inferior vena cava to certain cardiac stents, total hip implants, and surgical mesh without any clinical trials to ensure safety and efficacy.

Clearance of high-risk implanted devices through the 510(k) exemption, which has occurred in 21 percent of cases, is particularly dangerous because it is based on two potentially false assumptions—first that the predicate device is safe and effective and second that the manufacturer's claim of "substantial equivalence" ensures that the new device is at least equally so. In truth, devices cleared through the 510(k) pathway were simply grandfathered in without any clinical trials, so there is no guarantee that either the predicate device or its follow-on device is safe or effective. In 1996, the US Supreme Court concluded that "since the 510(k) process is focused on equivalence, not safety, substantial equivalence determinations provide little protection to the public."[192]

Since 2009, the FDA has reclassified almost all previously un-classified devices—a move intended to ensure that high-risk devices will be labeled as such and subjected to the agency's premarket ap-proval process, requiring "scientifically valid" evidence. However, only a tiny fraction of such devices are subjected to clinical studies, and the FDA's definition of "scientifically valid" evidence includes "partially controlled" trials, the use of historical controls, case re-ports, observational data, and surrogate end points—the sort of data most experts understand to be often misleading.[123] Vinay Prasad, an oncologist and a nationally recognized expert on evidence-based medicine, said of the FDA's approval process, "[It] is so bad [that] some physicians I know privately call the device market the Wild West, where a company can still 'strike gold' and where it really doesn't matter if the product works to make patients feel better or live longer."[193]

Yet the Supreme Court ruling on preemption presupposes that the approval process is bulletproof and provides sufficient protection to the public. If that were the case, the FDA would not have to recall about eleven hundred devices annually. A number of recalls are "class 1" recalls, which, according to the FDA, means there is "a reasonable probability" that the recalled device could "cause serious adverse health consequences or death."

Individuals implanted with recalled devices face the difficult choice of undergoing surgical removal, with all its risks, or waiting it out with the worry that something might go wrong.

As devices become increasingly complex and invasive, the number of class 1 recalls has been rising year after year: in 2003, there were eight class 1 recalls; that number rose to 176 in 2013.[194] The number of the FDA's supposedly "stringent" processes of premarket approval, intended to ensure the safety of devices before they go on the market, has declined over the years, while the use of other pathways to approval or clearance has increased—pathways that require little if any clinical testing. This has occurred at the same time that implanted devices have become more complex by several orders of magnitude, with computer-driven, Wi-Fi-enabled devices programmed to electrically stimulate the heart and brain and devices that combine biologic products and drugs with high-tech gadgetry.

In 2001, the agency approved seventy-one devices via the PMA pathway; in 2005, the number dropped to forty-three. By 2009, only twenty devices were approved via the PMA pathway. During the same time frame, PMA supplement approvals rose, increasing from 641 in 2001 to 1,394 in 2009. So how did all these high-tech devices get on the market? In addition to the many 510(k) clearances, manufacturers can apply for a *supplement* approval when they alter an already approved device in a manner they say does not alter safety or effectiveness. There is also a so-called real-time supplement application pathway, which allows manufacturers to make a phone call to the agency to review the changes for approval, after which the agency will fax approval to the manufacturer.[195] In most instances these alternative pathways do not require clinical trials.

Of course the device approval process upon which the Supreme Court rested its preemption ruling is itself a thin reed, because only a tiny fraction of the highest-risk implanted cardiac devices that won approval under the PMA process were subjected to two randomized blinded trials.[15] And because only 16 percent of high-risk devices go through the original PMA process, the overwhelming majority of high-risk devices have never undergone a single controlled clinical trial much less the putative standard for drug approval: two randomized controlled clinical trials.[15, 190]

The VNS device is a poster child for the problems that arise when the public is forced to rely on the FDA's premarket approval process as an assurance of safety and efficacy. Even though the VNS device underwent two randomized (partially) controlled clinical trials prior to approval, the FDA's lax oversight both during and after the approval process is evident. The company was let off the hook regarding the possibility that the device causes deaths, which couldn't be definitively determined because Cyberonics failed to include a comparison group of patients treated with medicines only. Nor did the FDA demand such a comparison group.

In 1997, during premarket deliberations, when Steven Piantadosi, one of the FDA advisers, expressed concern about the seventeen deaths that occurred among the first one thousand patients—a number that was particularly alarming in part because patients had been implanted for only a few years at most—a Cyberonics representative assured the panel that the deaths were the result of sudden unexplained death in epilepsy (SUDEP). In other words, according to the company, epilepsy, the underlying condition, not the VNS device, caused the deaths. But Piantadosi continued to express concern, saying, "I'm still a little worried about the death rates that we are seeing…Should we be concerned by that?"[133]

FDA reviewer Ann Costello responded to Piantadosi by citing a study that showed a somewhat higher mortality rate from SUDEP among patients about to have brain surgery to treat particularly severe seizure disorders. W. Allen Hauser, a member of Cyberonics' scientific advisory board, was also quick to acquit the device, saying,

"I don't think that the sudden death is an issue specific to the device. It's a specific issue in terms of people with bad epilepsy."

There were reasons to doubt Cyberonics' claim of safety. The company used data from "worst-case-scenario" patients—those who were about to undergo brain surgery as a "last-hope option" to treat intractable seizures. But those patients often have well-defined risk factors that increase their chances of dying early, such as multiple grand mal seizures; and serious developmental problems. The VNS device was not being tested for use on people who experienced grand mal seizures: instead it was tested on individuals with partial seizures, which pose a lesser threat of early death.[196]

But something else made a comparison of Cyberonics' test subjects to "worst-case-scenario" patients unfair: all Cyberonics' potential test subjects were screened and excluded from clinical trials if they had serious conditions known to increase mortality, such as diabetes and heart conditions—or a serious seizure disorder causing two or more episodes of status epilepticus in a year. In other words, Cyberonics study patients as a group (who comprised a portion of the first one thousand implanted patients) were not as likely to be in the same high-risk categories as patients about to undergo brain surgery.

The only true way to know whether the VNS device was saving lives or killing people would have been to enroll a third group of test subjects in a medically managed group.

Piantadosi challenged the suggestion that the VNS device might decrease deaths from SUDEP by reducing seizures. Calling seizure reduction a surrogate marker for the desired outcome of reduced SUDEP deaths, he said, "I would emphasize again that short-term outcomes or surrogate outcomes don't always fully inform us about longer-term outcomes, and I am still a little bit uncomfortable with the death rate."[133]

Leaving the question of the VNS device's safety open while still approving it (albeit conditionally) shifted the burden of proof from Cyberonics to the public: patients would have to serve as unwitting test subjects to determine whether the device was safe. Of course, prospective patients weren't told that "the FDA is concerned about a high number of deaths among test subjects, and therefore the VNS device has been awarded only conditional approval, and full approval will only be granted when the agency determines whether it's safe." That might not have gone over so well. Nor did the FDA require the company to tell doctors or patients this in the product labeling. Had that information been provided, it's not clear how many patients would have opted for VNS implantation. It seems likely that at least some would have rejected the device had they known that accepting it was tantamount to offering themselves as guinea pigs.

Given the scant data on the VNS, it is possible that patients overall would have done neither better nor worse without the device. Policy experts generally agree that we could substantially improve the quality of healthcare and reduce costs if only we would do more research to determine what in medicine works best and for which patients. Giving patients care they don't need exposes them to untold harm and contributes to a growing mountain of wasted healthcare dollars. Michael Wilkes, a professor of medicine and vice dean of education at the University of California, Davis, says, "We don't like to acknowledge the uncertainty of medicine, either to ourselves or to our patients. But patients deserve to know when their doctor's recommendation is backed up with good evidence and when it isn't."

The failure of regulatory agencies like the FDA to provide Americans with the medical safety net they deserve and honest information about the devices to be implanted in their bodies has led to enormous costs in terms of wealth wasted, resources squandered, and lives lost.

Chapter Seven

REGULATORS IN CHAINS

AFTER THE SUPREME COURT ruling, Fegan's fight for himself was over. But that hardly slowed him down. If anything, the *Riegel v. Medtronic* ruling and the death of his own case fueled his determination to bring the problem of the VNS device to light. "There were still people out there being killed by this thing," he said.

Smoking a little more than his usual pack-a-day habit, he redoubled his efforts. He wrote to the Texas attorney general's office and to the state health department. He e-mailed officials at the FDA, along with every media outlet he could think of.

He felt like he was hanging on by his fingernails. It had been two years since he was hospitalized, and no one seemed to be taking his concerns about the VNS device seriously. Cyberonics continued to deny there was a problem. The FDA had done nothing. Politicians sent him form letters in response to his pleas for help, thanking him for his "concern." Then without any pretense of offering assistance, they put him on their mailing lists asking for campaign contributions.

On September 8, 2008, Fegan filed a complaint with the Texas Department of State Health Services. He asked the state investigators to look into the company's failure to report his near-death experience to the FDA. He told them about the Cyberonics representative who "danced all around" his question about whether the company would report the issue to the FDA and never gave a straight answer. He told them that Cyberonics had failed to report at least sixty deaths to the FDA and that the company was continuing to "keep the FDA in the dark." He even provided a Web link to warning letters from the FDA to Cyberonics citing their failure to report deaths.

The company had "no reason to be forthcoming with the FDA," he wrote. "The FDA is well aware that Cyberonics failed to report my life-threatening [experience]. All of my complaints to them have fallen on deaf ears. The Vagus Nerve Stimulator is killing people and the FDA is doing nothing about it. How many more people have to die before the device is removed from the market?"

When he didn't hear back from the health department, he wrote to the Texas attorney general on October 2, 2008, stating:

...748 VNS deaths have been reported to the FDA. Approximately 1/3 of those deaths list the cause as either "Unknown" or "Sudden Unexplained Death of Epilepsy." If my parents hadn't shown up that morning my death would have [fallen] into one of those two categories. Nowhere in those FDA reports do they lay blame on the VNS. I can't help but wonder how many VNS patients went through the exact same thing I did and never lived to tell their story...

He was surprised and hopeful when US Congressman Solomon P. Ortiz of Texas sent Fegan a copy of a letter that he had sent to the FDA, dated October 30, 2008, requesting an investigation into Fegan's concerns.

But the FDA's only response to Ortiz's inquiry was an undated letter from Lillian Jordan, the FDA's congressional affairs specialist, who informed Ortiz that there may or may not be an investigation, and if there was to be one, which they would not reveal, information about such an investigation would be available "pursuant to a Freedom of Information Act (FOIA) request, once the investigation is closed." Jordan helpfully provided Congressman Ortiz with the address and website where he could obtain a "handbook for submitting FOIA requests."

If the response from Ortiz's inquiry was a bureaucratic black hole, the response from the Texas attorney general's office was no response at all. That left the Texas Department of State Health Services, which responded a year later. On August 24, 2009, Lance Sindo, a Texas state drug and device investigator, began a three-day on-site investigation at Cyberonics' headquarters, in Houston. Sindo reviewed Cyberonics' records and met with four of the company's officers, including the head of regulatory affairs, the chief compliance officer, the vice president of quality, and the senior manager for clinical engineering and clinical technical support.

It would seem that an investigation into the relationship between the VNS device and asystole would require the expertise of a physician, yet not one doctor was involved: the state of Texas investigation was carried out by a handful of engineers and corporate officers. Each had an investment in the outcome. There was no independent patient representative or clinical reviewer. The Cyberonics officers could hardly be considered independent. And the company's determination of the "root cause" of Fegan's asystole was based on the report filed by Steven Parnis, the Cyberonics representative who'd attended Fegan's one-month follow-up visit at Bahamon's office. Parnis was not a physician, but, as a senior manager with the company, he may have had reason to portray the VNS as safe.

Fegan's hope that the state of Texas would investigate the cause of his asystole and whether other patients were at risk was misplaced. Sindo himself acknowledged that the state can only evaluate whether companies follow processes and procedures, such as filing reports with the FDA. What the state can't do, said Sindo, is "evaluate the relationship between a device and an adverse outcome."

Despite being disappointed yet again, Fegan still held out some hope. Perhaps he could open the door to a larger investigation by focusing on the company's failure to report his experience to the FDA, which was part of the state's mandate. Manufacturers are required to report serious adverse events and deaths within thirty days to the FDA. If a serious adverse event or death is "unexpected"— something not previously reported to FDA—they are required to file a report within five days, because such unexpected events could warrant a warning to the public or even recall of the product.

Eventually such a report in regard to the case of Dennis Fegan would surface. But as we'll see, there are troubling questions as to its authenticity.

★ ★ ★

With the rise and growth of the medical-industrial complex between the 1970s and the 1990s, it had become increasingly difficult for federal agencies charged with regulating healthcare to keep up with the intensifying demands and political pressures of their work. Making matters worse, in the decade prior to Fegan's hospitalization, the FDA increasingly became the defender of drug and device manufacturers' interests.

In healthcare, as in other areas subject to government regulation, the problem of "regulatory capture"—in which regulatory agencies habitually defend the interests of industry over the public interest— is a serious one. It occurs in part because many regulators leave agencies to take lucrative jobs in industry, providing valuable inside knowledge and government contacts to the businesses they once oversaw, including—sometimes—ways to circumvent regulations. It's not hard to imagine that this phenomenon could lessen the zeal with which government staffers monitor and challenge the activities of businesses, since they may well be (consciously or unconsciously) looking forward to the day when they, too, may benefit from the "revolving door" to industry. Why make too many enemies among the corporate executives whose ranks you may one day join?

When these dynamics become too powerful, a regulatory agency ends up being "captured," or controlled, by the industry it is supposed to police. Those agency staffers who are dedicated to protecting the public are often thwarted in their work by managers and agency heads who are most concerned about protecting corporate interests. In effect, while the agency continues to exist on paper and even to operate apparently as usual, it is chained, prevented from doing the tasks it was mandated to do by Congress and the American people.

It's up to cabinet officers and other high-ranking government officials to craft policies and make personnel decisions that minimize the danger of regulatory capture. Unfortunately, under "business-friendly" administrations, the opposite sometimes happens.

That has been the case with the FDA. The process began in earnest in 1968, when President Richard Nixon changed the position of FDA commissioner from civil servant to political appointee.[197] This was an historic move. Since US presidents are often beholden to the drug and device industry, thanks to their generous campaign finance contributions, it shouldn't come as a surprise that, since 1968, they have often appointed commissioners who are considered friendly to industry. There have been some notable exceptions: David A. Kessler, MD, who served from 1990 to early 1997, waged a ferocious fight against tobacco companies. But he was succeeded by a different breed of appointee.

Larry Kessler (no relation to David Kessler), the director of the Office of Science and Engineering Technologies at the FDA's Center for Devices and Radiological Health until 2009, says that when he first joined the FDA, in 1995, "I almost never felt that our decisions would end up on the desk of a congressman. A device company would occasionally claim things weren't going their way and a congressman would write to FDA and say 'What's going on?' and almost always if we explained, that would be it." But, he said, "things have become more and more political in general with an increased concern about what the Agency might hear from Congress." Kessler says user fees that device companies began to pay to the FDA in 2004 led industry to feel "empowered," thinking, "We're paying the bills and we want service for paying the bills."[198]

During the late 1990s and early 2000s, the revolving door between the FDA and the private healthcare sector began to spin faster than ever—in both directions. Industry employees and executives would leave their jobs to work for the FDA just long enough to promote policies preferred by their companies before returning to their industry positions.[197, 199–202] The agency is further kneecapped when politicians, most of whom are beholden to industry, intervene to change unwelcome rulings by agency scientists.

Dan Troy made history in more ways than one when President George W. Bush appointed him on August 20, 2001, as lead counsel for the FDA.[183] Troy's appointment was the first time that this key position was filled by a political appointee rather than a civil servant. It was Troy who penned the friend-of-the-court brief in support of the preemption doctrine in the *Riegel* case.

This was a dramatic change in traditional FDA policy. Troy's predecessor, Margaret Porter, a career civil servant, had strongly supported consumers' right to sue, because, she said, "even the most thorough regulation of a product such as a critical medical device may fail to identify potential problems presented by the product." She decried the "harsh implications of foreclosing all judicial recourse for consumers injured by medical devices" under preemption.[183]

The US Supreme Court cited Dan Troy's amicus brief as a contributing factor in its ruling on *Riegel v Medtronic*.[182] Under the preemption doctrine, although some courts allow suits to proceed if a device is considered "misbranded" or "adulterated," suits are preempted as long as a properly labeled device functioned as intended. In other words, if a device hasn't exploded or broken apart, and is continuing to function, any side effects are the patient's problem—and the patient can't sue. Because the heart-rhythm disturbances and asystole that Fegan experienced were side effects of a VNS device that was functioning as intended, Fegan was told by Winckler that he couldn't sue Cyberonics, thanks to the preemption ruling.

Even when devices do explode or fall apart, industry has another way to evade responsibility. If manufacturers can't find something about a patient to blame, they blame the doctor, calling it user error—which is precisely what Medtronic did in Riegel's case, a case the manufacturer won by claiming that the cardiologist filled the balloon beyond the recommended pressure.

Dan Troy's background prior to being named lead counsel for the FDA offers some insight into his priority: protecting the interests of industry rather than the well-being of the public. He was working for the law firm then known as Wiley Rein & Fielding, in Washington, DC, suing the FDA on behalf of drug and tobacco companies, when Bush appointed him. Troy's other clients included Pfizer, which paid $350,000 to Wiley Rein for Troy's services. Troy became best known for his involvement in the landmark Supreme Court ruling that the FDA doesn't have the authority to regulate tobacco.

Bush received substantial funding from drug and device companies and his family had ties to the industry: Bush Sr. was on the board of directors of the pharmaceuticals company Eli Lilly.

Bush had his own reasons to select Troy. In 2000, Lilly lavished $1.6 million on politicians—82 percent of which went to Bush and the Republican Party.[203] Bush needed to protect his benefactors, and Troy was a natural ally.

After joining the FDA, Troy asked lawyers representing drug and device manufacturers to inform him of lawsuits against them so the agency could help in their defense. He said, "We can't afford to get involved in every case—we have to pick our shots," but to ensure that the companies would get Troy's assistance, he told them to make their case "sound like a Hollywood pitch."[183]

Congressman Maurice Hinchey of New York charged Troy with a "pattern of collusion" with drug and medical device manufacturers, saying that the FDA had "corrupted its mission to protect the public health" and that Troy "is aggressively intervening against the public on behalf of drug companies and medical device manufacturers." He also told Congress that it was "the first time in history that FDA's Chief Counsel is actively soliciting private industrial company lawyers to bring him cases in which FDA can intervene in support of drug and medical device manufacturers."[183]

Undeterred, Troy persisted in his proindustry activities. After resigning from the FDA in November of 2004, he became a partner at the law firm Sidley Austin, where from the Washington, DC, office he "principally represented pharmaceutical companies and trade associations," according to his bio on the website of the pharma giant GSK, where he is now senior vice president.

The preemption ruling supported by Troy has created a curious double standard: individuals can still sue drug makers, but they can't sue device makers.[192] This is in large part a result of the different eras in which the two industries rose to power and came under federal regulation.[204] In 1938, the drug industry, while powerful, had not grown into the multinational behemoth it is today and was unable to forestall the 1938 Federal Food, Drug, and Cosmetic Act, passed in the wake of the 1937 sulfanilamide–diethylene glycol disaster, which caused 106 deaths.

The act stated that no "provision of State law" would be invalidated by the amendments except upon a "direct and positive conflict."[205] This meant that even if the FDA approved a drug, the public had recourse in state courts, and lawsuits were not "preempted" by prior FDA approval.

The medical device industry, on the other hand, didn't come under regulatory control until 1976, with the passage of the Medical Device Amendments. By then, device manufacturers had morphed into multinational corporate giants that gave massive campaign contributions to politicians and deployed armies of lobbyists on Capitol Hill. As such, they were able to achieve important concessions in the 1976 amendments, including a provision that laid the groundwork for preemption, which was confirmed by the *Riegel* ruling.

Dan Troy's career and his support for the *Riegel* ruling exemplify the problem of regulatory capture, but regulatory capture doesn't happen only under Republican presidential administrations. In 2009, President Barack Obama appointed Margaret Hamburg as FDA commissioner. Hamburg, a multimillionaire, was a board member of Henry Schein, Inc., one of the world's biggest medical device distributors, at the time of her appointment. She had to divest financial holdings worth in the vicinity of $1 million in order to assume the position of commissioner.[206, 207]

Hamburg made some positive changes during her tenure. For example, she helped usher in a plan to use unique device identifiers (UDIs) to improve the tracking and safety of medical devices. But she took several positions favored by industry, including a plan to loosen conflict-of-interest rules, thus making it easier for industry representatives to sit on panels that advise the FDA about certain drug and device approvals. When Hamburg made her proposal, industry representatives had already swung the vote on advisory panels, allowing drugs with deadly side effects to remain on the market, including the birth control pill Yaz, which caused an increase in strokes compared to other birth control pills.

By contrast, independent experts who have expressed concerns about individual drugs or devices have been charged with "intellectual conflicts" and excluded from FDA panels. In November of 2004, the FDA barred adviser Curt Furberg from serving on the panel considering the safety of a class of pain-relieving medicines known as cyclooxygenase-2 (COX-2) inhibitors.[208] Prior to the panel meeting, Furberg had been quoted in the *New York Times* as saying that "Bextra is no different than Vioxx, and Pfizer is trying to suppress that information." (Both drugs belong to the same class, COX-2 inhibitors.) The FDA cited his statement as evidence that he wasn't "impartial."[209] In the end, the advisory panel vote was closely split, but Bextra was withdrawn from the market. Furberg's involuntary recusal was in contrast to the substantial numbers of experts with financial ties to the manufacturer of devices and drugs under review who are frequently appointed to FDA advisory panels.[210] If panelists with financial conflicts of interest had been recused from panels, such as the panel that voted to keep the birth control pill Yaz on the market, the vote would have been reversed and Yaz pulled from the market.[211–213]

Hamburg's recommendation to include more industry representatives on advisory panels caused a public furor, and she ultimately backed away from her position. But she did manage to push through rules allowing faster drug approvals, a move loudly applauded by industry.

The proclivity of presidents to name industry-friendly leaders to head agencies like the FDA shouldn't be surprising, given that politicians across the board increasingly rely on industry, especially the drug and device industries, to support their campaigns. During the 2012 presidential campaign, Barack Obama and Mitt Romney each received more than $19 million from the healthcare industry.[214] This was no departure from the norm: industry generally funds politicians on both sides of the aisle in order to curry favor with whichever candidate wins. All sectors of the industry get into the act. In 2014, the top two health insurance groups, Blue Cross Blue Shield and America's Health Insurance Plans, contributed $12 million and $9.2 million respectively to politicians. With the FDA reliant on budgetary support from presidents and congressional leaders who, in turn, depend on the healthcare industry for campaign money, it's not surprising that the agency should tend to be cautious about thwarting the plans of companies in the medical-industrial complex.

The FDA depends on corporate support in other, less widely known ways. It receives money from industry through the Prescription Drug User Fee Act (PDUFA), passed in 1992, and the FDA's Center for Devices and Radiological Health (CDRH) first began receiving direct industry funds through the Medical Device User Fee and Modernization Act (MDUFMA) of 2002. The device center also receives support for its programs indirectly through the virtually unknown Reagan-Udall Foundation, which "advance[s] the mission of the FDA by advancing regulatory science and research."[215] The foundation received more than $4.1 million in 2013 from drug and device manufacturers. Overall, 43 percent of the FDA's budget and 28 percent of the CDRH's budget come from industry user fees.[216]

According to a November 2012 report by Partnership for Public Service sponsored by Pew Charitable Trusts, "large sums" of money from drug and device companies "in many ways influence how the FDA will spend the money," thereby forcing FDA officials to "deal with current political realities." The authors concluded that those realities were affecting the number of people hired for new drug reviews as well as the timelines for reviews and approvals, which in turn have "distorted the structure of the FDA's workforce, creating the potential for expertise gaps."[217]

In other words, money to speed up approvals was forthcoming. Money to tighten up safety...well, that wasn't on the agenda.

FDA review times of high-risk devices are indeed faster since 2006. And industry funding not only speeds up the approval process, it also may be playing a role in ensuring that devices win approval. During fiscal year 2015, the FDA approved 98 percent of all high-risk device applications.[216] That's up from 86 percent in 2014.

It's not hard to point to specific examples of how regulatory capture plays out in the daily operations of an agency like the FDA. Numerous devices have been pushed through the FDA approval process with scant to no evidence of benefit or safety. Some have been deadly. The Sprint Fidelis defibrillator, which was implanted in hundreds of thousands of heart patients, was recalled in May of 2009, after it was found to misfire, seriously harming and killing numerous patients. John Mandrola, a cardiologist, said that when the device misfires most patients can tolerate the first 750-volt shock, but "almost no one can tolerate multiple shocks...after a second or third shock, anxiety...progresses quickly to near terror."[218] The harm is particularly disturbing given that, according to cardiologist Rita Redberg, "many, if not most" defibrillator implants are unnecessary.[14]

Other cases include the 1999 recall of the ProtoGenmesh, which was implanted during surgeries to support internal organs and tissues, after it was found to have caused bowel perforations, bleeding, and at least seven deaths.[219]

In 2008, the FDA cleared Menaflex, a device made of bovine cartilage and used to repair or replace a torn or damaged knee meniscus. The maker of Menaflex, a New Jersey–based company named ReGen, had pushed for fast-track clearance through the 510(k) pathway, claiming their device was "substantially equivalent" to surgical mesh. FDA scientists rejected the company's request three times, concluding that Menaflex wasn't effective, that it caused multiple adverse events in 42 percent of patients, and that the device wasn't substantially equivalent—after all, surgical mesh doesn't have to stand up to pounding as it would in a joint like the knee, nor is it made of cow cartilage.[141, 220]

Faced with rejection, ReGen did an end run around the FDA scientists. They approached their friends in Congress, after which three New Jersey Democrats met with then FDA commissioner Andrew von Eschenbach, who in turn complied with several of ReGen's requests, including that he put Daniel Schultz, then director of the CDRH, in charge of a new hearing (Schultz was widely perceived as a friend of industry). Eschenbach also required that the agency bar its own scientists from the hearing (ReGen charged that they were "biased") and agreed to appoint five outside experts recommended by ReGen to the new panel. In fact, Eschenbach not only named Schultz to head the review, he also named Gerald E. Bisbee Jr., who was ReGen's president and CEO at the time, to the panel.[141]

Eschenbach was so eager to assist ReGen that FDA attorneys had to tell him to cut a comment he made in a draft of a letter to the company because it could get the agency in hot water by revealing the favoritism shown to the company.[141]

Unsurprisingly, the new panel Eschenbach appointed overruled the FDA's own scientists and approved the device without explanation.

In 2010, on the heels of a congressional investigation launched by Senator Chuck Grassley, the FDA acknowledged it had yielded to political pressure, and the agency rescinded its clearance of Menaflex.[221] But ReGen appealed the agency's decision, and on September 26, 2014, an appellate court ruled in favor of ReGen. Ivy Sports Medicine bought out ReGen and now sells Menaflex as the Collagen Meniscus Implant (CMI).[222]

Donna-Bea Tillman, former director of the Office of Device Evaluation, was criticized for caving to political pressures in the Menaflex case. She left the agency after seventeen years, and in a talk sponsored by the University of Michigan Medical School, she coached device entrepreneurs on the nuances of the 510(k) pathway:

> [The] 510(k) is the pathway that most people who are developing new medical devices are likely to run into, and it is the pathway that requires you to identify a predicate device, which is a legally marketed device, [to] show that your new device is substantially equivalent. So that's what you need to do. And it's kind of interesting because what I find is that a lot of my clients and a lot of people developing new devices, they want to say, "Oh, my device is novel and it's new and there's nothing else like it out there." And that is absolutely *not* what you want to tell FDA, because you want to be able to say to FDA, "Well, yes, even though I may have some new features or a slightly different technology, it's substantially equivalent to what's already out there." Because that's what enables you to go through this 510(k) pathway, which is a lot less costly and expensive and burdensome than going down the PMA pathway.[223]

This double-edged sword of being different while simultaneously claiming substantial equivalence has created a logical loophole exploited by industry, which the Institute of Medicine concluded can't be repaired. Despite the IOM's 2011 recommendation to eliminate the 510(k), there has been no movement in that direction. Indeed, industry has been pushing for even fewer restrictions on their march to market.[224]

In chapter 4, I described how Cyberonics managed to win approval to market the VNS device to treat depression despite the unanimous protests of nine scientists on the FDA's review panel who considered this approval inappropriate and ill advised. We know what happened in this case because the scientists involved chose to take a public stand—a stand that cost several of them their jobs.

In 2008 and 2009, "the FDA Nine" wrote to Congress, and then to President Obama, complaining about corruption at the agency and political interference.[225] In their letters, they cited the Menaflex and VNS cases as examples of the way corruption and political influence at the FDA were trumping science. The scientists also described other questionable FDA rulings. For example, they said that FDA scientists had unanimously recommended against approval of a digital mammography machine. But their recommendation was overturned following a call from Congressman Christopher Shays, who represented the district where equipment for the device is manufactured, to Dr. Donna-Bea Tillman, then the director of the Office of Device Evaluation. (Shays told the *New York Times* that he called the FDA simply to demand a final decision—not to force approval.)

The FDA Nine also cited approval of a CT colonography device after scientists declined to approve it. One of the Nine, Julian J. Nicholas, MD, PhD, concluded that there was no "demonstrable evidence" that screening with CT colonography would reduce deaths. He also warned that the device wasn't safe, because a single examination delivers a radiation dosage equivalent to eight hundred chest X-rays—a dose that could cause cancer in between one in seven hundred and one in one thousand screened individuals.[226]

When Nicholas refused to clear the device, FDA managers indicated they would clear it anyway. Nicholas then asked another medical officer at the FDA, Dr. Robert C. Smith, to independently review the device. Smith agreed and concluded that "the device should not be cleared," and that if cleared, "it would pose a serious public health risk."

When it became clear that the FDA was going to approve the device regardless, Nicholas and Smith contacted various legislators, journalists, and a whistle-blower organization in an attempt to forestall approval. When their concerns were published in the *New York Times* and other media outlets, General Electric, manufacturer of the colonography device, complained to the FDA, suggesting that that the FDA Nine were guilty of releasing "proprietary and confidential" information.

Claiming that they needed to monitor any leak of proprietary information, FDA managers spied on the scientists' private and encrypted Yahoo and Gmail accounts and, according to their whistle-blower lawsuit, "stole the whistleblowers' confidential communications" with their attorneys, members of Congress, and the US inspector general regarding "allegations of serious wrongdoing by the agency."

Eventually the FDA fired four of the FDA Nine, and FDA managers asked the Office of the Inspector General (OIG) to initiate criminal proceedings against the FDA Nine. Despite repeated requests by the managers, the OIG declined, each time stating that the FDA Nine had the right to raise their concerns with Congress and the media.

Despite the ruling by the OIG, FDA managers and the agency's director of the Center for Devices and Radiological Health (CDRH), Jeffrey Shuren, continued their secret spy operation against the FDA Nine for at least two years. But Shuren took the spying to another level: despite the OIG's assurance that the FDA Nine's communications with Congress and the media were protected, Shuren filed criminal charges against at least two of the FDA Nine, charging that they may have leaked confidential information to the *New York Times*.

The FDA Nine countered that the FDA actions violated their constitutionally protected communications with Congress.

After learning of the spy operation, and after six of the nine suffered harassment and retaliatory firings, those six scientists filed suit against the FDA and its managers, including Margaret Hamburg and

William Maisel, for interfering with their First Amendment right of free speech. The suit was dismissed in September of 2014 by US District Court judge Reggie B. Walton, who ruled that although the spy operation was "troubling," the plaintiffs had failed to exhaust administrative remedies prior to filing suit.

Despite the agency's claimed concern that the FDA Nine were leaking commercially protected information, FDA managers never demanded that the scientists stop their communications or return the documents they shared with Congress or the media—undermining the managers' claims that the information was actually proprietary.

The FDA's spying produced no intelligence regarding leaked proprietary information. Instead, according to Stephen Kohn, executive director and attorney with the National Whistleblower Center, who is representing the scientists, they followed the officers' whistleblowing activities, using screen shots and minute-to-minute recordings of each keystroke on their computers.[142]

One of the FDA Nine, Robert C. Smith, the former radiology professor at Yale University who was a device reviewer at the FDA until July of 2010, when his contract wasn't renewed, told the *Washington Post,* "Who would have thought that they would have the nerve to be monitoring my communications to Congress? How dare they?"

Michael Carome, deputy director of the public-interest organization Public Citizen Health Research Group, urged the FDA in 2012 to tighten its lax oversight of medical devices. Citing device failures such as a "surgical clip designed to clamp off arteries that pops off, causing patients to bleed to death, and [a type of] artificial hip that shreds metal fragments…causing extreme pain and limited mobility," Carome said that the "massive lobbying effort" by the device industry was threatening the public health.

One might think that regulators would be moving to close loopholes and tighten restrictions on industry in order to stem the flow of faulty products that reach the market. Unfortunately, the evidence suggests that the FDA is working hand in hand with industry to dismantle even the weak protections currently in place, a problem that has greatly accelerated with the Trump administration.

The history of entanglements between industry and the top brass at the FDA should make the recent scandals unsurprising. In 2005, the FDA commissioner at the time, Lester M. Crawford, mysteriously resigned just two months after being confirmed. His resignation may have been tied to a Justice Department finding that he had illegally withheld information about his financial ties to companies that the FDA regulates.

Daniel Schultz, CDRH director from 2004 to 2009, resigned in the middle of the Devicegate scandal. Schultz was sharply criticized during a Senate investigation by Senator Chuck Grassley for overruling FDA medical officers' unanimous recommendation not to approve ReGen's Menaflex knee device and Cyberonics' VNS device for the treatment of depression. AdvaMed, a trade association for device manufacturers, had praised Schultz for ensuring that the CDRH obtained a constant flow of industry funding.

Jeffrey Shuren, the current director of the CDRH, became acting director in September of 2009. Shuren is so cozy with industry that he had secret meetings with AdvaMed to shape the 21st Century Cures Act, which lowers the bar for evidence needed to approve devices. In December of 2015, Inside Health Policy, an online news service, obtained e-mails and documents under the Freedom of Information Act revealing that Shuren and AdvaMed "met regularly during the legislative process and that the agency and the device lobbying arm had jointly written legislative text." The news service wrote that during a meeting on August 7, 2015, AdvaMed "thanked Dr. Shuren and the Center for Devices and Radiological Health team for meeting with AdvaMed regularly during the legislative process for getting the 21st Century Cures Act passed."

The 21st Century Cures Act, signed into law by President Obama in December of 2016, severely curtails FDA oversight of the medical device industry. The act, says Diana Zuckerman, president of the National Center for Health Research, instructs the FDA "to help drug and device companies get their products on the market more quickly. Unfortunately, it does that by loosening and lowering the very scientific standards that have made FDA approval the gold standard for countries around the world."[227]

The act includes provisions that allow the use of what industry likes to call real-world evidence, which could include individual case reports, observational studies, and even speculation based on post hoc subgroup analyses.[228] But such low-level evidence is unreliable and has misled doctors and the public in the past—sometimes with disastrous results. Consider the use of high-dose chemotherapy for breast cancer. For decades doctors subjected women to highly toxic doses of chemotherapy and bone marrow transplants in the belief that they were saving lives. But that belief was based on case reports and observational data. When five randomized controlled trials were finally completed in 1999, it was clear that the brutal treatment was no more effective than conventional chemotherapy and caused far more devastating side effects, including heart failure and death.[90]

The act also includes a provision that allows manufacturers essentially to approve certain of their own devices without FDA input. Here's how it works: Device manufacturers currently must win FDA approval when they make changes to high-risk implantable devices. Under the act, manufacturers will be able to hire a third party to determine whether their "quality system" is adequate. Once certified, manufacturers will effectively be able to decide whether their own devices are safe and effective.

The assumption that third-party certification, paid for by industry, will protect the public ignores recent history. Third parties hired to evaluate their paymasters know that return business is dependent on satisfied customers—a dynamic that played a central role in the run-up to the great recession of 2008, when financial analysts, hired by investment bankers, gave high marks to toxic investments. Similarly, evaluators who are financially dependent on the device manufacturers they are evaluating may be tempted to ensure repeat business by not finding too much fault with their paymaster's products. And if a third party's evaluations are critical, companies can simply hire a more compliant evaluator. This arrangement assumes a degree of honesty and fair play that has not been the trademark of device makers. For example, consider just a few selected fines levied against Medtronic:

- in 2008, Medtronic was ordered to pay $75 million for false claims regarding the need to hospitalize patients treated with its bone-cement product;
- in 2011, Medtronic was fined $23.5 million for paying kickbacks to doctors to encourage implantation of its pacemakers and defibrillators;
- in 2012, Medtronic agreed to pay $85 million to settle a class-action lawsuit regarding illegal corporate promotion of bone-graft material for off-label uses;
- in 2014, the company was fined $9.9 million for paying kickbacks, again to doctors who implanted the company's pacemakers and defibrillators (kickbacks included free flights to events, used as "free vacations" by some doctors, along with "gifts of wine and alcohol" and "trips to strip clubs");
- in 2015, Medtronic was fined $2.8 million for selling its spinal-cord-stimulation device, which "lacks evidence of clinical efficacy," without FDA approval;
- in another 2015 action, the company was fined $4.4 million for labeling imported devices as "made in the United States" so it could sell them to the US military;
- in 2016, Medtronic admitted that over the course of five years

it failed to report more than one thousand adverse events to the FDA related to infuse its spine-implant device (the company said the reports were "misfiled" and the failure to report was "unintentional"); no criminal or civil penalties have been assessed to date.[229]

Medtronic is not an exception; similar rap sheets exist for many if not most companies. In 2007, Johnson & Johnson was fined $84.7 million by the Justice Department for paying kickbacks to doctors who implanted its artificial hips and knees. In 2011, it was fined $70 million to settle civil and criminal charges that it bribed doctors in Europe and Iraq to sell artificial joints as well as its drugs. Biomet, Inc., was fined $6 million for paying kickbacks to doctors to promote use of its bone-growth stimulators in 2014, and in 2012 the company paid nearly $23 million for giving kickbacks to foreign doctors.

The list of companies forced to pay civil and criminal fines is extensive—not only in terms of the number of companies involved but also in terms of the number of repeat offenses committed by each company. Concealing harmful side effects, paying kickbacks, and promoting off-label use of devices continue unabated. Fines are simply the cost of doing business and are listed as potential or anticipated costs in each company's Security and Exchange Commission filings.

Nor do these actions have adverse consequences for the companies' CEOs or bottom lines. As of early 2015, Omar Ishrak, CEO of Medtronic, earned $1.5 million in base salary and enjoyed a total annual compensation package of $39.5 million. The average salary and compensation package for the CEOs of the eighteen publicly traded device companies in the US was $1.3 million and $15.4 million respectively as of 2015.

Civil and criminal fines don't necessarily slow sales of worrisome devices. Patients and doctors often remain unaware of court rulings and FDA actions, instead relying on professional publications, which can be blissfully upbeat when company-paid researchers publish reports that accentuate the positive while eliminating the negative.

Medtronic, which moved its headquarters from Minneapolis to Ireland in 2015 in a "tax inversion move," announced that sales that year of its spinal implant, Infuse, were climbing fast, reaching $740 million globally, beating Wall Street estimates by $20 million. Medtronic, the second-largest device manufacturer behind Johnson & Johnson, saw its fiscal-year 2016 revenues soar to $30.24 billion, up from $16.18 billion in 2012.

★ ★ ★

The revolving door between private industry and the federal government is one major cause of regulatory capture. Direct pressure on scientists and civil servants from politicians is another: in many cases, a phone call to an FDA manager from an important member of Congress is enough to cause an FDA head to overrule a disapproval by the agency's medical officers. But sometimes sterner measures are needed. There have been times when Congress has used its power of the purse to thwart regulatory agencies by simply threatening to defund them.

In the early 1990s, Richard Deyo, a prominent spinal surgery researcher, and his colleagues incurred the wrath of the North American Spine Society (NASS) by publishing several studies suggesting that spinal-fusion surgery is often ineffective and sometimes harmful. Industry backlash was ferocious.[230] The NASS, which is heavily funded by the companies that make the plates and screws used in spinal-fusion surgery, attacked Deyo and his sponsor, the federal Agency for Healthcare Policy and Research. The NASS mounted a full-frontal lobbying campaign targeted at key members of Congress, who in 1994 voted to eliminate the agency's entire budget. Only intensive efforts by the American Medical Association and the American Hospital Association restored 75 percent of the original budget. But the damage was done: the agency was prohibited from issuing comparative effectiveness guidelines and was renamed the Agency for Healthcare Research and Quality (AHRQ)—the word *policy* notably removed from its name.

Now the AHRQ outsources research to a mix of academic and contract research organizations. One of the AHRQ research groups, RTI International, based in Raleigh, North Carolina, received approximately $161 million of its $807 million funding in 2014 from "commercial and nongovernmental" sources, according to a spokesperson for the institute. Another, Duke Clinical Research Institute, receives approximately two-thirds of its $331 million annual revenues from industry.[231]

Since Congress cut AHRQ's funding by 25 percent and stripped it of its independent research capabilities, spinal-fusion operations have increased dramatically, says Deyo, and new surgical devices have proliferated. Despite the increase in surgery, there is little evidence of benefit for many patients: three of four randomized controlled trials in Europe found "very little advantage over rigorous rehabilitation for back pain due to worn-out disks," said Deyo. The long history of industry influence and intimidation, he says, has left the device-approval and surveillance systems in shambles.[230]

In the absence of tough, independent regulation, some device problems have become so egregious that manufacturers and the FDA have been forced to issue recalls. There have been recalls for defibrillators that caused continuous shocks, pacemakers that failed to fire, surgical mesh that bred infection, and bone-growth products that have caused paralysis, breathing trouble, and death. Recalls of malfunctioning or poorly designed devices disrupt the lives of hundreds of thousands of people who suddenly have to decide how to handle the danger within them. One study, published in the journal

PLoS One, found that in 2004, there were two recalls of stents with design flaws that had led to breakages that could cause perforations, heart attacks, and death, affecting a total of 96,000 people. In 2007, the FDA issued a recall on the Sprint Fidelis defibrillator, affecting 268,000 individuals worldwide, 172,000 of them in the US. In 2011, the agency recalled 79,000 more defibrillators because of failures that also led to serious injuries and deaths. A 2010 recall of DePuy metal-on-metal artificial hips affected 90,000 individuals; a 1999 recall of pelvic mesh affected tens of thousands of women. In 2013, 33,000 inferior vena cava filters had to be recalled when it was found that instead of preventing clots from reaching the heart, they actually caused clots.

Of course no device is perfect. Even the best devices will invariably cause harm and death for some. Lifesaving pacemakers have killed some individuals; artificial hips have poisoned some patients, causing everything from the death of surrounding tissue to heart and thyroid failure. The question is not whether a device ever causes harm but whether the benefits are expected to exceed the harm in a defined population.

Unfortunately, there is little hope that the FDA will serve as a stalwart defender of public health against potential abuse by device manufacturers as long as it is subject to the long arm of industry. Over the years, the agency's independence has been grievously compromised, leaving patients like Dennis Fegan virtually unprotected from the harm that oversold and poorly vetted medical devices can do.

Chapter Eight

THE POWER OF ILLUSIONS

In 2008, Dennis Fegan came across the online transcripts of the FDA's Neurological Devices Panel meeting held on Friday, June 27, 1997 to consider approval of the VNS device. Fegan was excited. Perhaps this document would shed some light on the mysterious process by which the company had earned the right to unleash its unproved technology on the American public.

Levering Keely of the FDA staff called the meeting to order at 10:11 a.m., a late start because of a bomb scare at the building. He said it was important to "push things along," given that a number of the participants had flown in from other parts of the country and had their return flights booked based on the time the hearing was scheduled to end—4:00 p.m.

Harold A. Wilkinson, professor of neurosurgery at the University of Massachusetts, served as the chairman. Seeming a bit unfamiliar with his role, he asked FDA staffers a few times how to approach procedural matters. Wilkinson was one of ten voting panelists. The others were all neurosurgeons or neurologists, with one exception:

Steven Piantadosi, a professor of oncology and biostatistics at Johns Hopkins, was specially trained in methodology (the ways in which clinical studies are designed and interpreted).

Other participants included five Cyberonics representatives (four of whom were doctors), a lawyer for Cyberonics, one "consumer representative," and three FDA staffers. Five members of the public—patients, their family members, and advocates—were also present as scheduled speakers; they would lead off the panel's discussions.

The first patient, Tim Fabian from Binghamton, New York, told the panel that before he had his VNS device implanted he had "10 to 15 seizures a day," but since his device was activated, in January of 1996, he said, "I have had no seizures."[*]

The next speaker, Paulette Machara, chief executive officer of the Epilepsy Foundation, said the VNS would be the "first device treatment option for epilepsy" that might help the "nearly one in three" patients with epilepsy whose seizures aren't completely controlled by other means. She added her concern that seizures can be "life-threatening" and that medicines for epilepsy can be "harmful to a developing fetus."

Machara was followed by Nancy Jean, who told the panel that following implantation with the VNS device, her son, Albert, not only had fewer seizures but also went from being behind in school to winning an academic achievement award and becoming more independent. She concluded, "Albert has been given back his life thanks to the stimulator."

Robert Cassidy told the panel that before he was implanted with the VNS device he had two to three seizures a month despite taking three medicines for his seizures. After implantation, he said his

---

[*] Fabian testified eighteen months after his device was activated. It is impossible to know whether he continued to be seizure-free, because he is deceased and a close relative was unable to give any information.

seizures dropped to "close to nonexistent," and he was able to take just one medicine instead of three. He told the panel, "The VNS changed my life."

The last member of the public to address the panel was Patricia Kroboth, whose son, George, was just seven months old when he had his first grand mal seizure. Over the years, despite multiple medicines and brain surgery, his seizures persisted, and Patricia was running out of hope, until, she said, "I picked up the newspaper one day and was immediately drawn to a picture of a teenage boy [who] looked exactly like George. The boy had a vagus nerve implant." Kroboth was overjoyed at the prospect of the VNS device, which meant, she said, "For the first time, there would be no powerful drugs and all of their side effects.... There would be no invasive surgery, with all of the complications that become a parent's worst nightmare."

George underwent implantation in April of 1995 at the age of twenty-three. Kroboth said, "George was not a rapid responder. Slowly, over the coming months, she added, "we started to see a decrease in the numbers of seizures.... In the past two months... we have twice seen a period of 19 days with no seizure activity. The last time we could make that claim, George was 9 years old." The number of drugs he took was reduced from five to three. Kroboth concluded, "The implant doesn't need to stop all seizure activity to change someone's life."

The five testimonials from the floor were powerful; even Fegan had to admit that. And they were all positive. Reading the transcript carefully, he tried to understand the gap between the testimonials, the evidence Cyberonics presented that persuaded the panelists to approve the device, and the deaths that continued to mount in the MAUDE database. After the testimonials, the scientific deliberations began. Fegan's training as a paramedic gave him some familiarity with the terms used by the FDA panelists, but because he had no special training in medical research or how studies were constructed, he found it slow going. He read and reread the statements of the FDA advisers, and when he saw a red flag, a statement of concern, he homed in on the references, looking for meaning and hard numbers.

It was during this painstaking process that he got a real shock: although some test subjects did have fewer seizures, between 20 and 33 percent of patients had *more* seizures. He was dumbfounded. It seemed that after implantation with the VNS device, roughly as many patients had more seizures as had fewer seizures.

How was Cyberonics able to claim that a third of patients benefited from the device if a similar number of patients did worse? Could it be that the entire basis of Cyberonics' business—the possible reduction in seizures provided by its VNS device—was based on a mere illusion?

★ ★ ★

One of today's leading experts on medical illusions is Dr. Jerry Hoffman—the same Jerry Hoffman we met in chapter 2 as a young medical student who aroused the ire of Eugene Braunwald through a bit of irreverent humor. Over the course of his three and a half decades of doctoring, and as a professor of medicine at UCLA, Hoffman has learned why doctors are so often flat-out wrong about diseases and their treatments. As a former director of the UCLA Doctoring Program, he has taught countless medical students and resident physicians, many of whom say he has influenced them more than any other doctor. Doctors from around the world seek out Hoffman for his insight and advice. He has lectured on several continents and held visiting professorships in Paris, Tokyo, London, and Santiago.

I attended a lecture given by Hoffman in New York City in June of 2011, when he addressed an audience of physicians at Bellevue Hospital. Tall, white-haired, and wearing thick glasses that magnify shiny dark brown eyes, Hoffman looks part elder statesman and part absentminded professor. His clothes are slightly rumpled, and bits of his hair stand out at right angles to his head.

He begins his talk at Bellevue by focusing not on the body or on any particular treatment but on language. "Words in medicine often have a different meaning than they have in ordinary English usage," he says. "And how we use language is really important." As an example, Hoffman draws our attention to the word *significant,* used in so many studies and marketing campaigns. "In common English," Hoffman says, "this word means something entirely different than what it means in statistics—in the larger world out there, if something is described as 'significant,' we all understand that it's important." If a drug or device is reported to have a "statistically significant" effect, many of us might assume that means it works. In statistics, though, "significant" is, well, less significant. As Hoffman explains, when a study finds a difference that is "statistically significant," it implies absolutely nothing about whether the difference is important. It simply means that the finding *probably* wasn't attributable to the play of chance.

Hoffman cites a study in which use of a certain drug "significantly" decreased the temperature of patients with fever. "Even if we buy that the observed drop in average temperature, from 101.0 to 100.7, wasn't due to chance and 'really' was due to the drug—is that *clinically* important? Does it mean patients will feel any better or have a better outcome? What is statistically 'significant' may or may not be clinically meaningful."

Hoffman then asked his listeners to think a little more deeply about the role of chance, saying, "This, too, is an area where we can easily be misled. We often assign meaning to a chance occurrence in our life when it seems too strange to have happened without a reason. Most of you have surely had an experience where just yesterday you thought about someone you hadn't seen for a long time...and then today he called! You think that's too strange to simply be a coincidence—there must be some deeper reason! But extraordinarily rare events actually happen all the time. How many people do you think about, if only for a second, every day...the vast majority of whom *don't* call?" For every million "one-in-a-million" events that *could* happen, the vast majority do not...but one of them will. We just don't know which one of these rare possibilities that is—and are extremely surprised when it does happen.

Using games of chance to illustrate his point, he said, "Any one person's chance of winning the lottery is virtually zero, but *someone* ends up winning it every time. Waiting for a particular extremely unlikely event is almost certain to be disappointing. But of the infinite number of extremely unlikely events out there, some—an infinite number, actually, if you want to be mathematically precise—do actually happen."

Hoffman's example helps to explain the medical illusions created by the five patient and family-member testimonials in the FDA hearings. Each was powerful in the telling, and each was resoundingly positive. While individual patient stories are important and can lead doctors to new discoveries, they need to be understood in context. If a treatment works fabulously in only ten out of a million patients, but those ten are the only ones to testify, we would get a distorted picture of that treatment. In the same way, if the VNS device works really well for most patients and causes problems in very few, then Fegan's quest to have it removed from the market would be akin to a patient's family demanding that penicillin be taken off the market because a family member died of an allergic reaction to the drug. Context, and the overall comparison between harm and benefit, are essential.

Unfortunately, all the statistics in the world can be a poor cousin to the power of anecdote and testimonials. Studies show that doctors as well as patients fall under the sway of anecdote.[232, 233] While the glowing testimonials offered at the 1997 FDA hearing were impressive enough individually, the fact that all five testimonials, including one from the director of the Epilepsy Foundation, were positive might seem to suggest that there is no question about the safety and efficacy of the VNS device. But that would be an illusion.

One of the powerful forces driving illusions in medicine is money, which not only biases research design and reporting but also influences patient testimonials. The patients and family members who addressed the panel that day were not chosen at random from the entire pool of people implanted with the VNS device. They were not the injured, as Dennis Fegan was. Nor were they the family members of patients who died after implantation. Instead, each patient or family member was carefully selected. And their airfare, food, and hotel accommodations were paid for by the Epilepsy Foundation, which, as Paulette Machara, the foundation CEO, acknowledged, did receive funding from Cyberonics. After each member of the public spoke, he or she was asked, as required by the FDA, to reveal any financial conflicts. The disclosures were all exactly the same as this interchange between patient Robert Cassidy and the panel chair, Harold Wilkinson:

DR. WILKINSON: And again, your way was paid by the—
MR. CASSIDY: My way was paid by the foundation.
DR. WILKINSON: And not by the company.
MR. CASSIDY: Not by the company whatsoever.

This is routine at FDA hearings: the manufacturer of whatever device (or drug) is being reviewed pays a foundation or "patient group" in order to put its commercial message in the mouth of a seemingly independent third party. Then the third party, either alone or with the help of the manufacturer, selects patients to testify who will promote the product under review by the FDA. It's a well-worn path of high farce: industry effectively launders its money through third-party organizations, and everyone acts as if it isn't happening.[*]

The process is akin to Congress inviting only the winners of million-dollar lotteries to testify about the "benefits" of gambling. Losers are not invited. Selection is everything, and as the saying goes, "Dead men tell no tales." *What is not reported is equally as important as what is reported.*

This doesn't mean the patients were dishonest—not at all. They were the lottery winners, and they were honestly describing their good fortune. But whether a patient's good luck is indeed attributable to the device or to luck is another matter. While it's possible that the VNS device has led to improvement in a subset of patients, it's also possible that their improvement was the result of other factors altogether.

The play of chance, and our human desire to find meaning in whatever we experience, takes other forms that can mislead us. Hoffman described another example: "My very first patient as a student on the medicine service noticed a lump in his armpit while reaching for something in his closet. The lump was actually a lymphoma, and of course it had been there for quite some time. But since he first noticed it when reaching, he connected the two in a way that made sense to him—he was sure the lump meant that he 'must have strained something.' That allowed him to impose some

---

[*] According to Cyberonics' SEC 10-K filing for 1996–97, the company identified one of the "key elements" of its marketing strategy as providing "education and support of patient advocacy groups such as the Epilepsy Foundation of America." The Epilepsy Foundation's annual reports reveal that by 2013, Cyberonics had contributed hundreds of thousands of dollars to the foundation (between $100,000 and 249,000 in 2013 alone). Cyberonics' president and CEO at the time, Daniel Moore, was on the foundation's board of directors, and three additional Cyberonics executives were serving on the foundation's business advisory board.

sort of order and rationality on the world. In fact we all do that, all the time, and it usually helps us understand our experiences. But not infrequently it also leads us to conclusions that are simply wrong."

Like Hoffman's patient who connected the lymphoma under his arm with the action he was taking when he found it, patients who improve following implantation with a device are bound to believe the device caused the improvement. Yet studies show that a sizable number of patients with temporal lobe epilepsy (the form associated with partial seizures) undergo spontaneous remission. They simply stop having seizures for reasons unknown. More than half of 190 epilepsy patients who were followed for a mean duration of eleven years underwent spontaneous remission.[234] Another study, of sixty-four patients followed for a median of thirteen years, found that nineteen of them (31 percent) attained a five-to-fifteen-year remission and were able to remain off treatment without seizures.[235]

Another factor contributing to the illusion of benefit is the placebo effect. Patients will provide testimonials that they were cured of cancer by the laying on of hands or that coffee enemas cured their arthritis. It's not that these patients aren't honest—or didn't improve. In some instances, they improved dramatically. But the power of belief, chance timing, and the natural fluctuations of illness and spontaneous regressions that occur with almost all diseases—even some deadly cancers—can lead to potent illusions.

The placebo effect is no less powerful with implantable medical devices than with drugs. During the hearing to approve the VNS device, FDA adviser Piantadosi commented on the fact that one of the measures of benefit claimed by Cyberonics—the total number of seizures experienced before and after implantation—could not control for the placebo effect because test subjects knew they had the device and all believed they might benefit. A real demonstration of benefit could come only from a differently designed study involving a medically managed control group.

Another key to the prevalence of medical illusions is the fact that not everyone is using the same yardstick to measure results. As Hoffman told the physicians at Bellevue, the word *benefit*, like the word *significant*, has a meaning in medical research that is entirely different from its meaning in common usage, and that difference frequently misleads doctors and patients alike. When used in everyday language, *benefit* is assumed to mean *net* benefit. If someone says she made a financial investment that was beneficial for her, we understand that the return on her investment was greater than any charges or fees she paid.

That isn't the case in medical research, where benefits are defined and reported separately from harms. In some ways that's for a good reason. If a treatment is intended to reduce heart attacks, and it does so, but it also causes liver damage in some patients, there is no single outcome measure that can reliably capture the true picture of the treatment. But this approach has opened the door to manipulation by sponsors who may test multiple end points and use multiple measuring sticks, then report only the findings they like. Frequently the study design itself prevents the full picture from emerging.

Similarly, Cyberonics used an isolated measure of benefit to declare the VNS device a winner. They defined *benefit* as the percentage of test subjects who had at least 50 percent fewer seizures after implantation. As for test subjects with an increased number of seizures? Well, that percentage was simply ignored in the calculation of benefit, because that's not part of the company's definition of *benefit*, or effects caused by the device. Instead, individuals who had more seizures were listed in small print under side effects. In this way, Cyberonics could claim in promotional materials that approximately a third of individuals obtained benefit from the VNS device.

Hoffman cites another example that illustrates widespread misunderstanding about the word *benefit*. Deaths from cancer are typically reported as "disease-specific" deaths, meaning that the benefit of a screening program for lung cancer is measured by the decrease in lung cancer deaths after screening. At first blush, that seems reasonable. Isn't that what everyone wants to know, after all? Do screening and treatment for lung cancer reduce deaths from lung cancer?

But as Hoffman points out, relying on disease-specific mortality instead of overall or all-cause mortality completely ignores the potential dangers of diagnosis and treatment. Even if screening for lung cancer prevents some patients from dying of this cancer—and thus decreases the disease-specific mortality—we can't know if screening is worth doing unless we also know whether it leads to just as many or more patients dying because of the screening program, whether from an invasive diagnostic procedure, or from surgery, or chemotherapy, or radiation. And that's only mortality: we also need to compare likely harm and likely benefit in quality of life, not to mention cost.

Despite the common perception that screening can only be beneficial, there are many documented examples of overall harm from screening. Hoffman tells us about one of these:

In the 1970s a device was developed that could accurately detect neuroblastoma, a deadly cancer affecting children. The device, used to test the urine of infants and toddlers, could pick up the cancer at a very early stage, long before children developed any symptoms. However, the test was abandoned after it was discovered that babies screened with the test were actually slightly more likely to die than unscreened babies.[236–238] It turns out that many of the tiny early cancers that were causing no symptoms, and therefore were only detected by screening, were very likely to regress spontaneously—so no one would have known about them if the babies hadn't been screened. But because doctors and parents didn't feel comfortable doing nothing, they treated *all* babies—not just babies with symptoms who actually required treatment.

Unfortunately, the program led to the detection of so many of the early cancers that a great many children were exposed to the potential perils of surgery—from which almost none of them could possibly benefit, since almost all these cancers would have simply gone away by themselves. In the end, the number of lives saved by treatment was exceeded by the number of lives lost because of the screening program.

According to Hoffman, doctors frequently fail to fully appreciate how the benefits of a treatment change with the severity of the condition being treated. He explains the concept, which he originally described in "Overdiagnosis of disease: A modern epidemic," published in 2012 in the *Archives of Internal Medicine*:

> Imagine a new antibiotic; we'll call it "gorillacillin." The drug is so toxic that it kills ten percent of those who receive it—after all, it's a very powerful drug that is tremendously beneficial for patients with the dread disease, "infectiosis," decreasing death rates from fifty percent to twenty-five percent. Gorillacillin is less attractive, however, when only 20 percent of treated patients actually have infectiosis; the 10 lives saved among the 20 patients who would have died are completely offset by the 10 drug-related deaths among 100 patients treated.
>
> Now imagine that all 100 patients actually have infectiosis, but 90 percent were diagnosed by sophisticated tests performed despite the absence of the classic fearsome symptoms of infectiosis, "just to be sure"—such that precious few have the deadly form of the disease. Since virtually none of these 90 were at risk of dying, gorillacillin would save 5 of the 10 truly at risk, but by killing 10, it would cause net harm. Overdiagnosis inevitably means that many individuals are subjected to the potential harms of treatment while being afforded almost none of its benefits.

The example of gorillacillin is counterintuitive; it flies in the face of conventional "better safe than sorry" wisdom and our belief that catching something early is "a stitch in time." But with the new screening test for "infectiosis," a different and far larger patient population is treated—a population in which many patients will recover without any medical intervention. Exposing this far larger population to the harms of gorillacillin now *increases* the chance of death.

Illusions and misunderstandings like these go a long way toward explaining how a highly questionable device like the VNS can get approved and even become a widely accepted treatment.

Common marketing tactics used by device manufacturers take advantage of medical illusions to increase the allure of their products. One such tactic is the indirect suggestion of a health benefit that the device doesn't actually provide.

Cyberonics' promotional materials, videos, and website feature patients who say that thanks to the VNS device, they were able to decrease or stop their medicines—freeing them of drug side effects. The belief that they would be able to reduce or stop medicine attracted many patients to the device. During the FDA hearing, Patricia Kroboth said that what excited her was the chance to get her son off medicines. And Paulette Machara of the Epilepsy Foundation implicitly suggested that stopping or reducing medicines would be an advantage of the VNS device when she said that it would benefit pregnant women because it "wouldn't harm the developing fetus." Yet in clinical trials of the VNS device, patients did not reduce their medicines.

Another unsupported, but implicit, claim by advocates is that the VNS device would save lives. Since individuals with epilepsy are known to have higher death rates than the individuals without epilepsy, advocates have emphasized the death rate when they promoted the device. But far from saving lives—there was evidence suggesting that patients implanted with a VNS device might be more likely to die—evidence that led the FDA to grant it only conditional approval.

A careful look at Cyberonics' claims of benefit reveals something quite different from the rosy picture painted by the company. Cyberonics' claim was based on the percentage of subjects in studies E03 and E05 who had a 50 percent or greater reduction in their seizures over baseline (as measured during the twelve weeks prior to enrollment in the study).[120, 135] According to the company, 31 percent of the high-dose group in E03 achieved a 50 percent or greater reduction in seizures, while 13 percent of the low-dose, or sham group did the same. The difference between the two groups was the best indicator of benefit, since the sham group's benefit was expected to be due to placebo effect. In other words, only 18 percent (31 percent minus 13 percent) of test subjects achieved a 50 percent or greater reduction in seizures. Cyberonics claimed in promotional materials that one-third of patients improved (based, apparently, on the 31 percent who improved in the high-dose group). Regardless of whether one accepts the 18 percent or 31 percent rate of benefit, this means that 69 percent to 82 percent of patients achieved no benefit whatsoever from the device—and indeed, as Fegan discovered while reading Cyberonics' data provided to the FDA, *one-fifth to one-third*[*] *of individuals actually had more seizures.*

In study E05, Piantadosi noted, the number of seizures experienced by test subjects was "highly skewed," meaning that while some patients had fewer seizures, others had many more seizures— as much as 690 percent more. Piantadosi said the true measure of benefit should be median improvement, and in that measure E05 showed no benefit. But Cyberonics used a different statistical

---

[*] Cyberonics didn't use the same percentage to quantify increased seizures as it did to quantify decreased seizures, making exact comparisons impossible.

measure to claim a benefit, one that nonetheless teetered on the edge of statistical significance.

The effect of the VNS device on seizures was like what happens when you squeeze a balloon in the middle—it caused the balloon to become bigger at the top (representing patients with fewer seizures) but it was also a lot bigger at the bottom (representing patients with more seizures). Cyberonics was effectively reporting only the top of the balloon without reporting the bottom to make its claim that the VNS device benefited a third of patients.

There were a number of other problems with Cyberonics' study design. During deliberations, the FDA's Ann Costello remarked that the company's claim of benefit in the one-year extension phase of study E05 was eroded "by the fact that the patients were changing their medications during this period." Had improved medication management contributed to the marginal benefit? Costello's point is one that dogs many device studies: there is often no control group of patients treated with medicines only and *without* a device. Failure to include a medical control group has led to many unnecessary device implants, from elective coronary stent placement to inferior vena cava filters—both of which were found to offer little to no benefit over medical management.[129, 239]

By failing to include a medical management arm of the study, Cyberonics set up a win-win situation, because one arm was bound to do better than the other. If the high-dose group performed better than the low-dose group, that was a win, and if the low-dose group proved superior, it would be possible to say that the high dose was simply too high. (Note the company's language—the doses were "presumed" therapeutic versus subtherapeutic, thus leaving wiggle room for just such a claim.) The study design made it impossible for Cyberonics to lose.

Nor could safety outcomes be accurately assessed, because Cyberonics excluded patients from enrolling in the studies if they had medical problems such as lung disease, heart disease, peptic ulcers, or status epilepticus. Certain later studies supported by Cyberonics claimed to show that the device could reduce deaths, but it did so by comparing study patients, which excluded the sickest seizure patients, and compared their death rate to historical control groups making interpretation virtually impossible, since reaching back to death rates among patients in the past ignores a host of confounders: Were patients in older timeframes treated with less effective medicines than they would be today? Were they a different age group than patients selected for VNS implants? Is it possible that VNS patients did better simply because they were less sick to start with?

When a study was finally conducted, in children, that did include a medically treated control group, the positive results were reported in the publication abstract this way: "55.4 percent of patients had at least 50 percent reduction of seizure frequency" and "VNS has been proven to be an effective alternative in the treatment of pediatric patients with drug-resistant epilepsy." But one has to carefully read the entire text to find what the authors failed to include in the abstract, their table of adverse events, or their conclusion section: during the three-year study period there were no deaths among the seventy-two children treated with medicines only, yet among just thirty-six children implanted with a VNS device, there were two deaths—one occurring after an increase in seizures.[240]

Research shows that most busy doctors, if they get to read studies at all, only read the abstracts and conclusions. They rarely read, much less critically analyze, the data presented, which not infrequently contradict the researchers' conclusions.[155]

A further clue that the VNS device might not have any real efficacy was buried in the company's 1997 physician manual (Cyberonics did not present these data during the 1997 hearing). In a review of what happened after a patient's VNS device stopped delivering shocks because of battery depletion, of seventy-two patients, 15 percent had more seizures, while 58 percent had fewer seizures. In other words, patients were far more likely to do better rather than worse when the VNS device stopped working.[241]

Of course, for patients with debilitating seizures, it's understandable that they might grasp at the hope that they will be among the ones to have fewer seizures. As Patricia Kroboth said, "The implant doesn't need to stop all seizure activity to change someone's life." Nor did it need to reduce seizures in every patient. But, as when playing the lottery, patients can't know in advance whether they will be winners—or losers. And the cost can be far greater than the $40,000 price tag for the VNS device itself. By 2016, the MAUDE database held reports of nearly two thousand deaths among VNS patients, and according to Tomes's database, the actual number was far higher.

Jerry Hoffman's crusade to educate doctors about the prevalence of medical illusions suggests that physicians can be an important bulwark against the harm such illusions can produce. But there are limits to what individual doctors can do to protect their patients. Doctors such as Fegan's neurologist, Juan Bahamon, might be faulted for recommending a flawed device like the VNS. But they rely on industry to paint a clear and accurate picture of the products that pour onto the market annually. And Cyberonics' claims were not only positive, they also appeared to have been vetted by the FDA. Fegan doesn't blame Bahamon.

Doctors can't be expected to review and digest several hundred pages of FDA transcripts and complex statistical data for each drug and device they prescribe. Ultimately they rely on FDA experts to interpret industry-funded studies for accuracy. There simply are no truly independent sources of research in the US. Industry funding has extended its reach into every sector, from medical journals that present and interpret the research to universities and contract research entities that conduct the research to patient advocacy organizations that promote various treatments to medical education for doctors to the agencies that are supposed to protect the public interest—including the Centers for Disease Control and Prevention, the National Institutes of Health, and, of course, the FDA.

Even if doctors could find time in the day to read and digest thousands of pages of original research data, most have not mastered the art of critical appraisal, the interpretation of statistics, and medical research findings (also called methodology).

Part of the problem is that doctors are on information overload. By the time they graduate from medical school, they've had to memorize every nerve, bone, and muscle in the human body. They've been trained to regurgitate detailed information about cell structure and biochemistry, disease pathology and pathophysiology, and pharmacology. They have to learn myriad laboratory tests, both common and unusual, and they will be expected to interpret certain X-rays and CAT scans and be adept at performing ultrasound. They will learn a wide range of surgical procedures, and they will even be taught some complex statistical concepts and calculations, which they will forget shortly after they take their board exams. They will get credit for "knowing the literature," but rarely do they gain an in-depth understanding of the critical skills necessary to distinguish solid science from research-based "evidence" that is actually unproved if not clearly wrong, as is so often the case.

To test how well doctors understand basic statistical claims, 160 gynecologists were given all the data they needed to come up with the correct answer to a question about mammogram testing. They were told:

- the probability that a woman has breast cancer is 1 percent (prevalence);

- if a woman has breast cancer, the probability that she tests positive is 90 percent (sensitivity);
- if a woman does not have breast cancer, the probability that she nevertheless tests positive is 9 percent (false positive rate).

Then the doctors were asked: if a woman has a positive test on mammography ("positive" means she might have cancer), what is the chance she actually has cancer?

A. The probability that she has breast cancer is about 81 percent

B. Out of ten women with a positive mammogram, about nine have breast cancer

C. Out of ten women with a positive mammogram, about one has breast cancer

D. The probability that she has breast cancer is about 1 percent

The correct answer is C: out of ten women who test positive on a mammogram, only one will actually have breast cancer. Yet only 21 percent of the gynecologists answered correctly, which is slightly less than the percentage who might have answered correctly had they merely guessed. The authors wrote: "Disconcertingly, the majority of [gynecologists] grossly overestimated the probability of cancer, answering '90%' and '81%.'" Expressed differently, of the ten total mammograms that are positive among one hundred women, nine are false positives* and only one is a true positive.[242]

---

* This may seem counterintuitive, but because so many more women (99 percent, to be precise) *don't* have breast cancer than do (only 1 percent have it, because the prevalence is 1 percent), the false positive rate affects many, many more women (9 percent of the 99 percent), so the false positives far exceed the number of women who actually have breast cancer.

Without an understanding of how research studies are designed, carried out, and interpreted, doctors—just like patients—fall prey to deceptive claims.

Faith in biological plausibility rather than misunderstood statistics is a source of other medical missteps. For many years, doctors used a medical laser to perform "transmyocardial laser revascularization," a procedure in which they would burn tiny holes in the heart muscle of patients with angina, or heart pain, in the belief that the holes would fill up with new blood vessels that would help deliver oxygen to the heart.[243] The surgery had the requisite scientific-sounding name and the seductive allure of laser technology.

It was biologically plausible that the holes could trigger new vascular growth—after all, the heart builds new blood vessels (called collateral circulation) to bypass clogged coronary arteries. But as Jerry Hoffman has pointed out, biological plausibility should be clinically tested before deciding that a treatment will be successful.

It would be many years after the surgery was adopted before researchers discovered that the holes simply filled up with scar tissue. Despite this, 46 percent of patients declared that the surgery made them better and they had less angina. Yet tests showed there was no new vessel growth. The strong placebo effect, along with persistent, unfounded faith in biological plausibility, encouraged doctors to continue a useless intervention until reliable studies showed that the surgery caused a dramatic increase in deaths and the practice was deemed "obsolete."[244] As Steven Nissen, chair of the Cleveland Clinic's department of cardiovascular medicine, likes to say, "The road to hell is paved with biological plausibility."

A patient's hopes and beliefs can play a role in the placebo effect. Even seizures can have a subjective component in terms of perception and reporting—especially partial seizures, in which fleeting moments of mental blurriness assumed to be a seizure prior to implantation with the VNS device are instead interpreted as trivial forgetfulness (rather than a seizure) after implantation. Some patients in the Cyberonics studies reported that although they still had the same number of seizures, the seizures they had were "less strong."

The patients and family members who testified during the FDA hearing were telling the truth from their perspective, and it's possible that some benefited from the device, but it's also possible that they were benefiting from the normal waxing and waning of seizure disorders, the placebo effect, or even spontaneous regression. Was it possible that Robert Cassidy, who testified that after implantation his seizures became close to nonexistent, was among the one-third of people with epilepsy who eventually undergo spontaneous regression? And what of George, who went nineteen days without a seizure after he was implanted? After all, he went nineteen days without a seizure at age nine, many years *before* he was implanted.

One myth about the placebo effect relevant to the VNS device is the belief that it only applies to symptoms that are psychological in nature or origin. Yet several studies dispel that myth. For example, a study of pain medicine versus placebo in patients thought to have psychological or functional pain rather than active disease (such as peptic ulcer disease or inflammatory bowel disease) showed that individuals with functional pain, as well as those with organic diseases, responded to the placebo.[245] Other studies have found that malingerers and certain patients with psychological pain may need their pain for some reason and therefore might be less responsive to the healing effects of a placebo than patients with organic pain.

The placebo effect can extend even to care providers. One young health aide caring for a mentally handicapped patient implanted with a VNS device said that when she activated the patient's device with a magnet, the results were miraculous! The patient's seizures would stop immediately (although the device fires every three or five minutes normally, patients can use a magnet to activate the device, causing an extra shock, intended to abort seizures). When asked how long the patient's seizures usually lasted if his VNS device wasn't activated, the aide said about two to three minutes. On further questioning, the aide acknowledged that it would take her thirty to sixty seconds to reach the patient, get the magnet, and swipe the VNS device. Adding up the time it took to first recognize that her patient was having a seizure, the time it took to get to the patient and disengage the magnet from the patient's wrist, and the time it took (another thirty seconds to a minute) for the seizure to stop after the aide swiped the device, it wasn't clear that anything had been gained.

The aide had been told that the device would stop seizures, and she interpreted the events in a way that made sense to her.

As if oblivious to the concepts raised by Hoffman's lecture about the impact of language and the fact that the words *significant* and *benefit* are frequently misunderstood, the FDA seemed to ignore the results of a study that demonstrated the gap between statistical significance, as emphasized by Cyberonics, and *clinical* significance. In an apparently unpublished study mentioned in a single brief paragraph of the 212-page transcript of the FDA advisory meeting, panelists learned that when the researchers examined thirty-four "quality of life" measures, they found no benefit in thirty-one of the thirty-four measures,[133] hardly evidence that the VNS device was improving the lives of patients, because chance alone would ensure that at least a few measures would be positive.

The sum of Cyberonics' research data, stripped of the emotional sway of anecdote and the misleading presentation of "significant" findings of "benefit," added up to this: 18 percent of test subjects improved in the short term, most patients failed to improve, there was no—or questionable—benefit over the long term, some patients experienced substantial worsening, and a concerning number died.

When Dennis Fegan learned that a sizable portion of VNS test subjects developed more seizures after implantation, he wondered: *How does anyone know whether a patient is having a seizure or a near-fainting or fainting spell caused by the device as it stops or slows the heart? And if it's a seizure, how does anyone know whether it's triggered by the device itself?* Just as asystole caused by the VNS device could be mistaken for SUDEP, it was also possible that seizures caused by the VNS device could be mistaken for underlying epilepsy. Fegan was grasping the concept of cure as cause, a source of widespread illusion in medicine.

When Cyberonics attributed decreases in seizures to the VNS device but attributed increased seizures to the worsening of epilepsy, it ensured that cure as cause was excluded from consideration. The problem is far from unique to Cyberonics. Whenever researchers assume that improvements are the result of treatment and bad outcomes are the result of an underlying disease or condition, they are ignoring the possibility of cure as cause.

Separate reporting of benefits and harms is necessary, but here's where things get sticky: because industry gets to decide whether an adverse event is caused by a device or an underlying disease, manufacturers can categorize the adverse effects of their devices as problems of underlying disease, creating another opening for industry to exploit the word *benefit* in ways that undermine objective research.

Hoffman says that cure as cause is not uncommon and should not be a particularly surprising phenomenon. Medical interventions, including those that involve devices, invariably interfere with the same physiologic pathways or organ systems that give rise to a disorder—and it's easy to overshoot or further disturb an already disordered system. And when outcomes such as hip pain, suicidality, and seizures mirror the symptoms of the underlying disorder, it's easy to miss cure as cause.

The problem is common with devices as well as drugs. Stents, intended to open clogged coronary arteries and prevent heart attacks, can themselves cause clots and heart attacks. Surgical mesh, used to prevent urinary incontinence, can slice through pelvic tissues, causing incontinence. Metal-on-metal hip implants that shed cobalt into the surrounding tissues can cause tissue destruction, leading to worsening hip pain that is mistaken for worsening arthritis. Filters placed in the large vein leading to the heart to prevent clots from reaching the heart have been found to trigger clotting.[224, 239, 246]

This isn't to say that every bad outcome negates the overall value of a device. It is a reminder, however, that all medical interventions come at a cost—costs that should be fairly measured and honestly reported so that the public can decide whether the risks that come with a device are worth taking.

* * *

Nearly one hundred years ago, Sinclair Lewis's Pulitzer Prize–winning book, *Arrowsmith*, featured Max Gottlieb, a medical researcher who railed against institutions that betrayed objective academic inquiry in favor of profits. Since that time, academic institutions and government agencies have become far more deeply enmeshed with industry, and the marketplace has been celebrated as a driving force that delivers cutting-edge science.

Jerry Hoffman, who has spent decades studying the ways in which industry manipulates study design, interpretation, and physicians' perception, has linked widespread financial conflicts of interest to misleading medical claims. For many years, like Lewis's character Max Gottlieb, Hoffman's seemed to be a lone voice in the wilderness.

But in the early twenty-first century, others within the medical community began to take up the cause. In 2005, John P. A. Ioannidis, professor of health research and policy and director of the Stanford

Prevention Research Center at the Stanford University School of Medicine, wrote an article entitled "Why Most Published Research Findings Are False." The piece took the medical world by storm, becoming the most downloaded article in the history of the journal *PLoS Medicine*. Ioannidis focused on the statistical illusions that cause bad science, but he also wrote, "There may be conflicts of interest that tend to 'bury' significant findings."

Studies consistently show that industry-funded research tends to exaggerate benefits while burying or failing to publish negative findings. Richard Smith, former editor in chief of *The BMJ*, the venerable professional journal once known as the *British Medical Journal*, has called attention to the unreliability of research published in even the most prestigious journals, concluding, "Medical journals are an extension of the marketing arm of drug companies." Marcia Angell, former editor in chief of the *New England Journal of Medicine*, echoed the same judgment, writing:

> *Let me tell you the dirty secret of medical journals: It is very hard to find enough articles to publish. With a rejection rate of 90 percent for original research, we were hard pressed to find 10 percent that were worth publishing. So you end up publishing weak studies because there is so much bad work out there.*

When I spoke with Hoffman after his lecture at Bellevue, he was in a reflective mood. "I was given the task of addressing the topic 'Diagnostic Decision-Making: How Clinicians Think,'" he said. "But I always like to bring this back to something I believe is just as important, which is our role as professionals. Drug companies have a fiduciary responsibility to their shareholders. As doctors, we have a fiduciary responsibility to put our patients first. By relying on industry-funded studies, we're failing our patients. As professionals, we have a special responsibility to make independent assessments on behalf of our patients, and we can't allow ourselves to be compromised by financial conflicts of interest."

Hoffman has pounded away for years at the ways in which industry funding of clinical trials and individual doctors has undermined good medicine. He rattles off examples. There was the study of calcium-channel blockers showing that researchers who received manufacturer funding were more likely to interpret results as positive than researchers who didn't have manufacturer funding. In another case, researchers employed by the manufacturer of dioxin were less likely than independent researchers to identify cancer in the slides of rat livers.

Hoffman quotes the famous comment by author and political activist Upton Sinclair: "It is difficult to get a man to understand something when his salary depends upon his not understanding it." "But that is our responsibility," says Hoffman. "Our society rewards doctors with enormous prestige and excellent income, not to mention almost unchallenged professional autonomy. In return, our patients expect us to put their interests above our own. We cannot take money from industry with one hand and write prescriptions with the other and remain a profession."

Chapter Nine

THE QUEST FOR TRUTH

On April 15, 2009, I was writing for *The BMJ* when I received the first of what would become many e-mails from Dennis Fegan. I was just one of the "dozens and dozens" of journalists whom Fegan had reached out to.

It took a while for me to look into his story and to reach a decision about whether the claims he was making were credible and whether his was a story I wanted to report. First, I wanted to get all his medical records. In addition, I wanted to contact the doctors who had treated him. Then I wanted Cyberonics' account of the matter, and I wanted the FDA's version.

I recall clearly the day that I received copies of Fegan's medical record. I read his ER report, and then I saw the cardiograms— electrical tracings of his heart, which gave a compelling picture of what had happened to him. In nearly thirty years of clinical practice, working in ERs and intensive care units, I'd never seen anything like this: There was a lengthy flat line, far longer than a mere pause or a few missed beats. It was the sort of flat line that one sees only as patients are dying—or already dead. I could see why Larry Johnson, the ER doctor who tried desperately to save him, remembered Fegan above all other patients in his more than thirty-year career.

Dates would prove important in what happened next. In February of 2010, I asked Cyberonics to send me its records on Fegan. The company said it couldn't discuss his case without his permission. On March 4, 2010, I sent Cyberonics a copy of Fegan's written release, authorizing me to discuss his case. Then a surprising thing happened: six days later, on March 10, 2010, the FDA received a report about Fegan's hospitalization—a report dated nearly four years earlier, July 3, 2006. Why the FDA didn't receive the report until then is not clear. Cyberonics insists it sent the report in 2006, but the FDA marked the report as received on March 10, 2010, the same day it finally appeared in the MAUDE database.

The report itself contained a subtle clue about its likely actual date. The company listed the date of Fegan's hospitalization as "May 2006." While the medical record clearly gave the actual date of Fegan's hospitalization as July 2, 2006, there was one place that also (erroneously) listed the date as "May 2006," and that was a report filed by Dr. Juan Bahamon, Fegan's neurologist. This suggests that Cyberonics may have copied the date of the event from Bahamon's report, which would give the lie to the company's claim that it submitted its report on July 3, 2006, because Bahamon didn't file his report until November of that year.

Furthermore, both the report Fegan eventually filed on himself and the report filed by Bahamon were dated as received the same day by the FDA. The four-year delay from the time Fegan was hospitalized to the time the FDA received Cyberonics' report was in stark contrast to reports sent to the FDA by Fegan and Bahamon, which were marked as received the same day they were sent.

Fegan told me there was something else suspicious about their claim that it took the FDA four years to suddenly log the report by

Cyberonics: if Cyberonics really had written its report the day after he was hospitalized, why did the company representative, Steven Parnis, demur when he was asked, a month after Fegan's hospitalization, whether the company intended to file a report with the FDA?

But the central point was undeniable: as Cyberonics acknowledged in its written report to the FDA, "both the cardiologist and the neurologist believe that the reported events were caused by the stimulation of the vagus nerve."

Cyberonics, however, wasn't about to let the conclusion rest at that. Instead, the company went on, "Inderal had recently been added to the patient's medication regimen." This point was supposed to be an evidentiary bombshell. Cyberonics was suggesting that Inderal was the crucial factor in Fegan's asystole. The company spelled this out in an "issue report" dated August 23, 2006, about the "root cause" of Fegan's asystole. The report concluded, "At this time the exact cause of the cardiac related event is unknown. It is possible for the cardiac events to be related to the initial [sic] of Inderal."

About two months before he was hospitalized, Fegan had indeed been started on a low dose of Inderal, a drug that can slow the heart rate. But it's highly unlikely that Inderal was the cause of Fegan's asystole. Inderal belongs to the class of drugs known as beta-blockers, which can reduce the heart rate by slowing passage of the electrical impulses between the atria (the top chambers of the heart) and the ventricles (the lower chambers). When this effect occurs, it causes readily detectable and very specific changes in the cardiogram. When Fegan's heart was beating, it was entirely normal. There was no slowing. There were no changes in the passage of impulses between the atria and the ventricles.

Furthermore, Fegan had been on the medicine for two months, which was plenty of time for his blood levels to stabilize and for signs of any problems to emerge. None did. As his neurologist indicated,

Fegan began telling his doctors about his new symptoms *before* he was started on Inderal, suggesting that the VNS device alone was indeed causing the problem. Nor was it possible to explain how Inderal would cause his heart to stop at exactly the same three-minute intervals that the VNS device fired or why his problem ceased immediately when the device was turned off—and while Inderal was still in his system.

For all these reasons, the link between Inderal and Fegan's asystole seems tenuous at best.

The Inderal defense was especially curious: if the company believed that beta-blockers like Inderal could cause a potentially fatal reaction when used with a VNS device, why didn't it issue any warnings to the public indicating that taking beta-blockers after being implanted with the device might cause asystole? Stephen C. Karceski, director of clinical trials at the Weill Cornell Epilepsy Center, gives talks (paid for by Cyberonics) to patients and doctors about the VNS device, and when asked if he cautions patients about using beta-blockers after implantation, he replied, "No. Of course not."

Warnings are a double-edged sword. If companies make cautions widely known, patients and their doctors might be reluctant to use a device. On the other hand, if a warning exists, the company is off the hook for urgent adverse-event reporting and, perhaps even more important, in the case of devices, it may be protected from lawsuits. Nothing served to immunize cigarette manufacturers against lawsuits better than the warning on cigarette packages about the serious health problems that can be caused by smoking.

At the 2017 BIOMEDevice conference and exposition in Boston, Michael Drues, PhD, president of Vascular Sciences, gave a lively presentation to members of the medical device industry on "how to address risks you'd rather not draw attention to in documentation." Drues is a heavyweight in the field: he is a consultant to big-name device and pharmaceuticals companies as well as to the FDA, Health

Canada, US and European patent offices, and governmental agencies around the world. The audience listened intently as he described various ways to deemphasize the unpleasant side effects of medical devices. He started by telling them, "Not many people can play on both sides of the fence," but of course it is precisely his ability to navigate both sides of the fence that makes him a sought-after expert. He told the audience that presenting device risks in order of severity or frequency can draw attention to risks the manufacturer might not want to emphasize and suggested that because there is no rule about how to present risks in a submission to the FDA they should instead list them in random order—and by listing a lot of minor side effects, they could effectively bury the worrisome effects in a lengthy list.

By issuing cautions but making them easy to overlook and difficult to interpret, manufacturers have the best of both worlds. The cautions get them off the hook—much as the warnings on cigarette packages now immunize tobacco companies against lawsuits over lung cancer—and because few people know of the caution, sales aren't harmed.

Of course, Drues counseled conference attendees, some things are better left unsaid. He quoted Massachusetts politician Martin Lomasney, saying, "Never write when you can speak; never speak when you can nod; never nod when you can wink."

Cyberonics handled the issue of beta-blockers and "heart stoppages" by simply staying mum. The company all but ensured that no one would know about the issue—not patients, not doctors, not even its own paid experts. There is no warning in any of the physician or patient manuals indicating that beta-blockers in combination with a VNS device might cause asystole and, potentially, death. That would be a bad marketing move, because beta-blockers are so widely prescribed that it would certainly cut the company's profit margins. But what the absence of information about beta-blockers more realistically reflects is that Cyberonics never believed that the Inderal Fegan was taking was the cause of or significant contributor to his "heart stoppages."

Cyberonics' failure to identify the VNS device as the cause of Dennis Fegan's nearly fatal asystole was of a pattern with its stance on the safety of its VNS device. On March 15, 2010, Cyberonics' vice president of clinical affairs and quality, Bryan Olin, a statistician, wrote in an e-mail, "We do not believe, nor does the data support, that there is any evidence suggesting that it [the VNS device] causes death." Earlier that month he said, "We have received no reports of post-operative asystole related to the death of a VNS Therapy patient." If that were true, then Fegan's life-threatening experience should have triggered an urgent report to the FDA of a new and potentially deadly problem. That might have led to a warning to doctors and patients. But none of the several dozen doctors I spoke with was aware of any problem involving asystole with the VNS device.

Similarly, the issue of increased seizures caused by the device was neatly obscured by the company. In an e-mail dated March 6, 2009, Joseph Tartal, the FDA's technical branch chief, responded to Fegan's query about why increased seizures weren't listed as a complication of the VNS device. Tartal told Fegan that companies are exempt from urgent reporting requirements if the problem is "well known to the medical community." But it was far from well known.

This was the same exemption the company claimed about asystole—asserting that the side effect was indeed well known. As evidence, the company pointed to the physician manual for the VNS device, which states that during implantation and testing of the leads, "infrequent incidents of bradycardia [slowed heart rate] and/or asystole have occurred."[247] But the company also insisted that no serious problems occur once patients are implanted other than allowing that bradycardia can occur "among patients with certain underlying cardiac arrhythmias." In other words, unless the patient already has heart problems, no worries, a point it underscored in its 171-page physician manual.[248] The Cyberonics patient manual simply lists "heart rate and rhythm change" as potential side effects. But the broad and rather innocuous phrase "heart rate and rhythm change" could mean anything and is a far cry from an emphatic warning that patients might experience heart stoppages and possibly die. Nor could such a low-key statement buried in a 171-page manual ensure that the information was well known by patients or their doctors. It certainly wasn't on the front page of the company's website or in any of its promotional materials.

There was something else that undermined the company's claim that the problem was well known. I interviewed David Newman, ER physician and then director of clinical research at Mount Sinai Hospital in New York City, about the VNS device, and he was unaware of any training for ER doctors conducted by Cyberonics to educate them about the device or its effects on heart rhythm. So he called a Cyberonics representative to ask how frequently asystole occurred with the VNS device, and the representative said he'd never heard of such a case. He did say he'd "look into it." He never did get back to Newman.

An informal poll (a questionnaire I e-mailed to a group of emergency-room doctors across the country asking whether they had ever been given training by Cyberonics or educated about the VNS device) led to just over a dozen responses. None of the doctors said he or she had been approached by Cyberonics or been given information about the device—nor did any of them have the equipment necessary to turn off the device in an emergency. This is in contrast to manufacturers of pacemakers and defibrillators, which have provided toll-free phone numbers and training for ER doctors so they can handle emergencies.

Had Cyberonics spent time doing the same, it might have meant the difference between life and death for thirty-six-year-old Shelly Rae Wilhite, who called her sister, Bridgette Coleman, on a Friday evening to tell her that her VNS device was suddenly giving her shocks that were so painful she fell to her knees.[249] She said she'd see her doctor Monday morning, because only her doctor could adjust the device. Doctors in the ER didn't have the equipment or the know-how to handle the problem. But Shelly didn't make it to Monday. On Sunday evening, September 13, 2010, Shelly's daughter found her dead on the bathroom floor.

The company so frequently failed to include critical information in its reports to the FDA that the agency finally sent Cyberonics a letter on November 13, 2008, stating, "Many death reports do not include sufficient information to determine a cause of death.... Please make an effort as much as possible to obtain event information... to determine the relationship of the device to the event."

Unfortunately, nothing changed after this scolding from the FDA. The MAUDE database is filled with reports—like this one, dated July 7, 2015—providing virtually no information: "It was reported that the vns patient passed away on [date redacted] 2015. The cause of death and its relationship to vns are unknown. No further information relevant to the patient's death has been received to date."

Although it's impossible to conclude definitively from such reports what caused a patient's death, we know from Fegan's case that the device can cause asystole.

★ ★ ★

By the time Dennis Fegan solicited my help with his case, the already thin rope he was hanging his hopes on was rapidly fraying.

The Texas Department of State Health Services had closed its investigation into Cyberonics on August 26, 2009, with no finding against the company. Since the state didn't have the authority to investigate the cause of Fegan's asystole, the only thing it could do was determine whether Cyberonics had followed proper procedures, filed papers, and filled out required forms, including reporting Fegan's asystole to the FDA.[*]

Politicians had proved unable or unwilling to help Dennis Fegan obtain justice. The media didn't do much better. My own article "Watching Over the Medical Device Industry," published in *The BMJ* on June 23, 2009, included a discussion of device regulation and problems with the VNS device.[230] But it failed to prompt any action. I followed up with Congressman Ortiz's office, who at Fegan's request had asked the FDA to investigate his case, but Ortiz's office told me I'd have to contact the FDA. His office would release no information.

When I contacted the FDA, a representative initially told me the agency could neither confirm nor deny whether it had conducted an investigation. If I wanted anything more, I would have to file a Freedom of Information Act (FOIA) request. Furthermore, *if* there was an investigation (which, the agency reiterated, it was neither confirming nor denying), information about it would only be available via FOIA once the investigation was closed.

After I filed additional requests, the agency told me that it had "no information responsive to my request."[250] After even more pestering from me, the FDA told me the case was "closed via telephone." I requested notes from the phone call between the FDA and Congressman Ortiz, and the agency told me it had no notes and that the Office of Legislation at the FDA said it was not required to keep notes.[251] Finally, after more phone calls and e-mails, the agency sent me a single-page document indicating that it did, indeed, receive communication from Congressman Ortiz, but virtually everything

---

[*] On the latter point, the state's investigator, Lance Sindo, accepted the form the company presented to him as proof that it had submitted a report.

on the page was redacted. When I said I would file a FOIA request to unredact the page, the agency reversed itself. Suddenly the case was not closed (which would have made the information open to a FOIA request). Instead, it said, the case was still open, protecting any information from release under the FOIA.

The claim that an investigation is still open *eight years after Ortiz's letter* is strange at best. But what it adds up to is simple: eleven years after Fegan's experience, any information about an FDA investigation—or an answer to the question of whether there ever was one—is locked up so tight that even my FOIA requests have failed to unearth it.

★ ★ ★

When I began researching Dennis Fegan's case and the overall track record of the VNS device, I was startled to see so many deaths among relatively young patients during the twelve years the device had been on the market. I asked Cyberonics for the postapproval study data proving the device's safety, required by the FDA as part of its conditional approval. Conditional approval meant that if the company didn't prove the device was safe, the FDA could order it off the market. Cyberonics forwarded five studies to me.[252–256]

I read each study carefully and was surprised to find that not one of the five studies included any data on deaths.

I immediately contacted the FDA, thinking that surely it must have additional data to prove the device was safe. But the FDA sent me the exact same five studies Cyberonics had provided.

I figured I must be missing some piece of the puzzle. So I went back to Cyberonics and asked for any *unpublished* data it had proving the device was safe. A representative said the company had proved it was safe with the five studies that were accepted by the FDA. When I asked the company to send me the death statistics for each of the five studies, because the results were not included in the published reports, to my surprise, Cyberonics explained that it had no death data to provide because it *never collected death data for any of the five studies.* When I pressed the company about how it could claim the device was safe if it didn't even know how many implanted people had died, I was told that it *had* collected mortality data from the Social Security Death Index—but hadn't published the results. When I asked for those data on behalf of the medical journal *The BMJ,* Cyberonics refused to release its findings.[100]

I was stunned. Twelve years after the device was approved for epilepsy, the company hadn't collected death data for the five studies it submitted as proof of safety and wouldn't release the death data it did collect outside of the studies. I informed the FDA, assuming that the company would get slammed by the regulator for failing to collect death data on a device approved only conditionally because of the FDA's concerns about a "high rate of deaths." But the FDA continued to insist the device was safe. When I pressed the agency about this, it responded in an e-mail that it hadn't asked the company to count the number of deaths, instead it only required Cyberonics to *"characterize* mortality." I wondered: How does one *characterize* mortality without knowing whether anyone implanted with the device died?

I was beginning to feel as if I were in a Kafka novel.

Fegan's finding that nearly a thousand VNS patients had died in just over a decade raised an important question: Could it be that the VNS device reduced a surrogate marker (in this case, the number of seizures) but increased the number of deaths? Could anyone tell the difference between SUDEP attributable to epilepsy and asystole attributable to the VNS device?

No one could answer the question with any certainty. The FDA's MAUDE database appeared to be intentionally useless: it didn't collect data on the total number of devices in use, making it hard to know whether serious adverse events were one in a million or one in a hundred. Nor were the ages of affected patients included. If a ninety-year-old patient dies three years after having a hip replacement, that's one thing; if a twenty-three-year-old dies after a hip replacement, it could be a clue to a serious safety problem. Nor does the database include the *reason* a device is implanted. The FDA would have no way to know how many patients implanted with a VNS device to treat depression developed asystole, since it simply doesn't collect those data. In an apparent lapse, Cyberonics listed the cause of death for a patient who was given a VNS device for depression as "SUDEP." There was no mention that the patient was epileptic. If the device was causing sudden death (called SUDEP by the company) in patients without epilepsy, this would be important news, and would be additional evidence that the device, rather than the underlying condition, was causing fatal asystole.

Making matters worse, the agency ignored its own demand for safety studies, giving Cyberonics a pass when it first approved the device and then another pass when it failed to collect death data for any of the five studies it submitted to the FDA as proof of safety.

The FDA had closed its case on the matter, but I continued to search the medical literature for an answer. Eventually I came across a study claiming that death rates were "similar" between patients implanted with the VNS device and those without it—but once again, the claim was based on an historical comparison group— observations of previous patients.[257] Jerry Hoffman, the expert on how medical illusions distort our understanding of research, says the study can't provide conclusive evidence about the impact of the VNS device. "One basis for skepticism," he said, is that "even though the authors report that the number of deaths among 1,819 patients with a VNS was 'similar' to the average mortality in several older studies of patients with 'refractory epilepsy,' there's no way to know if these 'control patients' were sufficiently similar to the VNS cohort to make any fair comparison." The authors acknowledged that they didn't know critical details about the patients that would tend to drive mortality up or down independently of the VNS device. They didn't have information on the patients' ages, seizure frequency, or causes of their seizures—each of which can have a powerful effect on mortality. With regard to the study's methodology, Hoffman said, "The devil is in the details, and there are far too few details provided."

Without a fair comparison, it's impossible to know if apples were being compared to apples. Many early VNS test subjects were included only if they were deemed to be "healthy"; some of the studies specifically excluded patients with a host of illnesses. The authors said they relied on the study sponsor, Cyberonics, to supply the death reports, writing that they "had no reason to assume" the company didn't supply all relevant data, an assumption that ignores the long history of selective reporting of results by Cyberonics and by industry in general. But one thing was clear, they weren't claiming a mortality benefit—only that the device didn't make things *worse* in terms of mortality.

Even some researchers funded by Cyberonics have grown disillusioned with the company's claims. Christian Hoppe, a neuroscientist and epileptologist at the University of Bonn, in Germany, had initially written about the benefits of the device.[258] However, as he analyzed his subsequent research findings and that of other researchers, he concluded that "the VNS literature" is replete with "bad science."[259, 260] He and his colleagues conducted a study of "therapy-resistant patients" who were treated with the "best drug therapy" with and without the VNS device implanted and found that patients with a VNS device fared slightly worse than patients treated with only drug therapy.[261] Their finding was consistent with two studies conducted by different researchers that also found no seizure-control benefit of the VNS device compared to simple drug therapy.

Another researcher on a Cyberonics study who was disturbed by the company's questionable scientific methods is Howard Barkan, formerly adjunct professor at the School of Psychology and Inter-disciplinary Inquiry at Saybrook University.* Barkan served as the statistician on a Cyberonics cost-benefit analysis study of the VNS device. The company claimed that the study proved the VNS is a money-saving investment that reduces long-term costs associated with epilepsy because it helps patients control their seizures—a nec-essary claim in light of the $40,000 price tag.

But Barkan says, "There was a systematic bias in what [the] Cy-beronics folks did." When all the data were in, Cyberonics wanted to exclude a particular VNS patient from analysis as an "outlier." The patient had seized and had a car crash. The hospital bill was in the vicinity of $150,000, which made the cost-benefit analysis "not look so good" when the patient was included in the analysis.

Barkan "wrestled and argued for months" over the exclusion, fighting the company's decision "tooth and nail." Finally, seeing no end in sight, he says he agreed to have the patient excluded on the condition that the case would at least be reported in a footnote. The authors submitted the paper, and Barkan says he was told the paper was rejected for publication. He forgot about it until several years later, when he saw that the article had been published with his name as a second author.[262] Barkan was infuriated: not only had Cyberon-ics thrown out the one "outlier" patient, it also, he says, "knocked out a subset of deaths that they didn't like."[262]

Barkan insisted on having his name retroactively withdrawn from the paper.

In the end, however, the researchers on this Cyberonics-funded study got to decide whom to select in its research, whom to ex-clude, and when and where the results would be published. Two

---

* Barkan died July 20, 2016.

Cyberonics employees conducted the statistical analyses, and the company acknowledges in the text of the article that three patients considered "outliers" incurred high medical costs—and yet all three were excluded from the final analysis, making the VNS device look cost effective.* As a result, Cyberonics can honestly claim that, according to published reports, the VNS device works, is safe, and is cost-effective. Doctors who read Cyberonics-sponsored research reports would have no idea about the contrary evidence swept under the rug.

* * *

The brick wall that Dennis Fegan and I ran into when we tried to investigate the safety problems with the VNS device is not unique to that device or to its maker, Cyberonics. Real information about the safety of implanted medical devices is difficult to unearth—even for people in a position to know.

Consider the case of Steve Tower, an orthopedic surgeon who was implanted with a medical device himself and suffered terrible consequences. Tower was far better placed than most of us to know about the true benefits and harms of the device, yet even he didn't have the information needed to understand the truth.

Tower, who specializes in complex artificial hip replacements and repair, knew in 2006, after five years of progressive pain in his right hip, it was time for him to get a hip replacement. Artificial hips have provided significant relief to millions of patients worldwide, freeing them from pain, allowing them to be active, and improving their overall health and independence. The implants have, until recently,

---

* The researchers did conduct what is called a "sensitivity" analysis in which they analyzed one of the three "outliers" and concluded that it did not affect their overall findings.

been celebrated as "one of the most successful operations of the 20th century."[263]

Tower chose what he believed at the time to be the best artificial hip on the market: the ASR XL metal-on-metal hip, introduced by Johnson & Johnson's DePuy division the previous year. The device had been cleared for sale under the 510(k) pathway, which meant the company claimed its artificial hip was simply a modification of a device already on the market. No clinical trials were required.

Tower had his ASR hip implanted in March of 2006. He did well at first. He was able to resume his hobby of long-distance bike riding. But about a year after surgery, things began to unravel. The pain returned and became progressively worse—as bad as it had been before the implant.

Troubled, Tower began to wonder if the ASR hip, which contained cobalt and chromium, might be leaking the metals, which are known to cause intense local inflammatory reactions that can damage tissue.[264] He obtained a cobalt level on his blood: it was two hundred times higher than normal. He contacted the manufacturer about possible complications from cobalt, but he says DePuy's design surgeons, engineers, and field representatives reassured him, "No worries...cobalt is harmless." Besides, they said, no other surgeons were reporting similar problems.

Over the following two years, the pain became excruciating. Tower's hip joint would grate and squeak with every step. He began having problems with his memory, vision, mood, and sleep. He developed ringing in his ears, and he could no longer bicycle any distance, because he became breathless with exertion. An echocardiogram revealed that he was in the early stages of heart failure.

Finally, in November of 2009, Tower couldn't take it anymore, and he had the DePuy ASR XL chrome-cobalt parts taken out and replaced with a new ceramic-on-plastic socket. When his surgeon opened up Tower's hip, he discovered what looked like a crankcase of dirty automotive oil. The tissues surrounding the hip were black. His surgeon said some of the ligaments had turned to "mush." Tower had metallosis, a condition caused by metals that can produce local and/or systemic effects. Local effects, the sort seen by Tower's surgeon when he removed the ASR hip, include tissue death and the destruction of muscles, bones, and ligaments. Systemic effects include nerve damage, mental changes, thyroid disorder, vision and hearing problems, and heart failure.[264–268]

One month after Tower had his ASR XL hip removed, his cobalt level plunged, and his mood and memory improved. Within a year, his heart function had returned to normal. Although his hip continues to dislocate at times because of damage to his ligaments, he is now feeling better.

A few months after his own corrective surgery, a patient Tower had fitted with a metal-on-metal hip complained of systemic symptoms suggestive of metallosis. Tower found the patient's cobalt levels were high. Following removal and replacement of his patient's artificial hip, his symptoms resolved.

Tower immediately began trying to sound the warning bell about the ASR hips and metallosis—specifically cobaltism, the condition he had experienced. But to his surprise, he ran into a brick wall at every turn. In May of 2010, he published two case reports of metallosis, his own and that of his patient, in the state of Alaska's epidemiology bulletin.[269] But the limited readership of the bulletin meant that only a few Alaskan doctors would learn of the problem. However, the Centers for Disease Control and Prevention (CDC) expressed interest in publishing Tower's report in its own widely read and prestigious publication, *Morbidity and Mortality Weekly Report*.

Tower was "elated" by the CDC's interest, but then, at the eleventh hour, according to e-mails dated late July of 2010, the CDC pulled the article, saying it was told by the FDA that it shouldn't publish anything because the agency was "studying" the issue.

In July of 2010, DePuy/Johnson & Johnson announced that it was withdrawing the ASR hip from the market because of low sales.[270] Later, the company issued a recall of 93,000 ASR hips, saying only that there was a high failure rate—12 to 13 percent—within five years. That compared poorly with other types of artificial hips, which last an average of fifteen years or more. But it was worse than the company was letting on: internal Johnson & Johnson documents showed that a whopping 37 percent of ASR hips failed after 4.6 years, sixteen times the rate for other hip implants.[271]

Early descriptions of metal ion leakage from implants were published as early as the 1980s and '90s, yet the reports received little attention.[272, 273] When mandatory device registries, which exist in Australia, the United Kingdom, Europe, Canada, and Japan—but not in the US—began detecting serious problems with metallosis, European authorities issued recommendations for routine screening of patients with metal-on-metal hips.[274, 275] Still, as recently as 2010, the phenomenon remained relatively unknown in the US when Tower published his report on two patients.[269]

Tower's seemed to be a voice in the wilderness.

Had US doctors and the public been alerted to the risk of metallosis and cobaltism earlier, it's possible that other patients might have been spared injury. In 2010, a fifty-nine-year-old woman was admitted to a hospital with heart failure, puzzling doctors, because she had no known risk factors.[276] Extensive testing failed to reveal the cause of her condition, which continued to worsen despite treatment with multiple medicines. She lapsed into end-stage heart failure, requiring two implants—first a device to help her heart pump and then a pacemaker-defibrillator. Ultimately she required a heart transplant.

It was only after her heart transplant that she—and her doctors—

would learn about cobaltism associated with the ASR hip replacements. She had had both hips replaced with ASR implants several years earlier. When she was tested for cobalt, the cause of her heart failure was finally clear: her blood cobalt level was extraordinarily high. After recovery from her heart surgery, she had both hips replaced. Her cobalt levels fell, and she began to recover from her other symptoms of cobaltism, including thyroid disorder and fatigue. And the function of her new heart improved.

Even a few case reports in the medical literature are hardly adequate to warn doctors or the public about serious problems with devices. A fifty-five-year-old German man went from doctor to doctor seeking an explanation for the onset of strange symptoms, including near blindness, deafness, thyroid dysfunction, fever, and severe heart failure despite normal coronary arteries. It was only when he landed on the doorstep of Juergen Schaefer, director of the Center for Undiagnosed Diseases in Marburg, Germany, that he would learn the cause of his problems. Schaefer, a fan of the fictional television series *House,* which features a cantankerous and unconventional doctor who solves mysterious medical cases, recalled an episode of the show from February of 2011 about a woman who had similar symptoms. It turned out they were the result of cobalt poisoning. Schaefer learned that the German man had had a metal-on-metal hip replacement a year and a half earlier and found that his cobalt level was one thousand times higher than normal. Following treatment, including replacement of his artificial hip with a ceramic hip, his heart function improved dramatically. Unfortunately, he had minimal improvement in his vision and hearing.[276-278]

When the FDA told the CDC not to publish Tower's reports because it was "studying" the problem, it was presumably to be "sure" there was a problem before alarming the public. But reports of possible adverse events involving medical devices are crucial to uncovering dangers. Clinical trials conducted for FDA approval often use limited numbers of test subjects and are thus too small to detect serious adverse events, which is why the FDA itself describes the value of its MAUDE database as an opportunity to identify "red flags." Recognizing a red flag can lead to a call for study to determine whether such reports represent a fluke or a genuine threat.

The question then is: What is to be done during the period after a red flag appears but before definitive studies are completed? It would seem rational to alert the public, adding the caveat that studies are pending so people can decide for themselves what steps to take. It's unlikely that patients already implanted would needlessly have their artificial hips surgically removed—or that surgeons would do so without evidence of a problem. But for individuals who have symptoms, the information provided could be important and could help their doctors know what to look for—and that might just save lives.

Tower's evidence of a possible link between cobaltism and hip replacements was important and worthy of publication. Yet Tower was shunned on multiple fronts as he sought to get the information out to doctors and the public. His report was delayed by a medical journal whose subsection editor and peer reviewers had extensive financial conflicts of interest. When the FDA finally decided, in 2012, to appoint an advisory panel for metal-on-metal hips, William Maisel, deputy director for science and chief scientist at the FDA's device center, turned down Tower as a panelist, referring him to James Swink of the FDA's Medical Devices Advisory Committee, who told Tower that panelists had to be nominated by industry or by the American Academy of Orthopaedic Surgeons (AAOS).[279]

Unfortunately, there is reason to doubt the impartiality of the AAOS. Like medical journals and conference organizers, professional medical associations often take large sums of money from industry. Industry money, lavished on every sector of healthcare, creates a feedback loop that encourages publication of positive messages about devices, while reports of harm remain relegated to the sidelines. Like other medical associations, the AAOS is supported by manufacturers who pay handsome fees to promote their wares at the association's annual conference.[*] Besides the institutional conflict of interest, many individuals in leadership positions at the AAOS have extensive ties to industry.

In the end, on January 17, 2013, more than two years after Tower tried to bring the problem to public attention, the FDA issued a "safety communication" in which it acknowledged that metal-on-metal hips could cause metallosis, which could lead to thyroid disorders, mental and nerve disturbances, psychological problems, vision and hearing problems, and heart failure.

By November of 2013, Johnson & Johnson had set aside $4 billion to settle lawsuits involving the DePuy metal-on-metal hips.[280]

In 2016, a careful meta-analysis (a study of multiple studies) of death rates among hip-implant recipients was published. The researchers found that patients with metal-on-metal hip implants were more likely to die early than individuals implanted with other types of artificial hips.[281] The two study sponsors were the Leiden University Medical Center, in the Netherlands, and the FDA.

Although DePuy stopped producing ASR hips in 2010, it had another product, the Pinnacle hip, which went on the market in 2002, and although the Pinnacle hip includes metal-on-metal implants, it remains on the market as of 2016. However, in March of that year, a Dallas jury awarded $502 million to a group of patients who said DePuy hid the Pinnacle's design flaws, which led to early failure and metallosis.[280]

Steve Tower says the ASR XL hip is implanted in only 10 percent of the one million patients who have with metal-on-metal hips,

---

[*] A spokesperson for the AAOS told me the "specific dollar amount is proprietary information."

which leaves nine hundred thousand patients who are also at risk—and an even greater number of patients with metal-on-plastic hips who may also be subject to metallosis. Tower wants to see patients protected through systematic screening programs like the ones now recommended in Australia and the European Union. Currently, routine screening in the US is not recommended.

* * *

Douglas W. Van Citters walks through a series of laboratories on the leafy campus of the Thayer School of Engineering at Dartmouth. The labs are collectively referred to by some doctors as the Dartmouth "device morgue." Van Citters, a tall man with a friendly manner and a boyish face, is associate professor of engineering and co-director of the college's Biomedical Engineering Center for Orthopaedics. He, his colleagues, and his students are on a constant quest to determine why and how devices fail.

As he walks through the labs, Van Citters points to some of the sixteen thousand medical devices that he and his colleagues have examined. They are sent to the morgue by doctors and hospitals from around the country.

The devices, which were once implanted in living humans, are now housed in museum-like displays and boxes. Each device has been explanted (removed) from a person—living or dead—for a variety of reasons. Some released metals that changed their human owners' muscles, hearts, or brains. Some broke into pieces. Some just stopped working. Each device has been sent to the morgue for analysis so the researchers can understand what went wrong, and in some cases, to understand what was right.

Van Citters stops beside several attractive wooden tables topped with glass enclosures that display dozens of explanted hip joints of various shapes and sizes. Some are plastic. Others are ceramic or metal. One particularly dubious-looking device has tiny bits of visible bone still attached. Like the other devices, this one is labeled with an identification number, below which is written: 22 YRS IN VIVO.

Another display reveals a large human thigh bone sliced open longitudinally. Protruding from the top of the bone is a gleaming artificial hip composed of a solid metal ball atop a long swordlike metal shaft that pierces the center of the thigh bone and extends through its marrow. What happened to the human owner of the thigh bone is a mystery. Van Citters is careful not to say too much. Confidentiality is maintained at the morgue, and only identification numbers are affixed to devices—no names.

Van Citters is the engineering equivalent of a forensic pathologist who conducts autopsies to determine the cause of death of murder victims. Many of the devices come from the Mayo Clinic, which keeps close tabs on device failures in hopes of avoiding future problems. Van Citters says his lab conducts testing not only to detect problems but also to enable the design of better devices by motivating "basic science research in tribology,* corrosion, materials, biomechanics, and so forth."

In certain parts of the lab, it's hard to hear Van Citters's voice over the roar of machines of various sizes and shapes that whir and grind, pump and rotate, as they shake, pound, and hammer away at their captive devices. Connecting the whirring machines is a dizzying network of clear tubing through which various chemical concoctions pass, bathing the devices in the numerous decay-inducing fluids that they might be exposed to in living humans.

Engineers examine micron-thin sections of devices with microscopes and even an electron microscope, searching for clues to material breakdown and corrosion. Oxidation is a particular curse. One

---

* Tribology is the study of surfaces in relative motion as well as the effects of friction, wear, and lubrication.

doctor who sends explanted devices to the morgue is Stephen Tower, the orthopedic surgeon. Van Citters and Tower share a mutual respect. They consult each other on things that have gone wrong and on the ways in which devices can be improved in order to avoid future failures.

Around 2015, visitors from the FDA came to Dartmouth for an "Experiential Learning Program." Van Citters says interested parties, whether lawyers or industry, can be invested in certain findings, but he says he tries to remain neutral, "like Switzerland," without advocating any particular position. He deals in numbers and hard science—not opinion. If a device has a defect, he'll point it out. If not, if some other factor is at play, he'll call it that way. In the meantime, the flaws he finds help him to develop materials and designs that are resistant to the problems he sees.

The quest for truth about the safety of medical devices is an inherently challenging one. Medical science is ever changing, human biology is enormously complex, and the factors involved in tracing cause and effect can be almost unlimited. Unfortunately, under the current healthcare system, the quest for truth is further hampered by the willingness of researchers, medical journals, and regulatory agencies to serve the interests of powerful corporations—even when the health of patients is put at risk.

Chapter Ten

WHEN MONEY TALKS

THE PROBLEMS THAT PLAGUE the medical device industry reveal a troubling pattern of financial kickbacks, perverse incentives, and institutional conflicts that too often give short shrift to the needs and safety of patients. The case of Infuse, a spine implant, offers a number of similarities to the VNS story.

In 2009, Kathleen L. Yaremchuk, chair of the Department of Otorhinolaryngology–Head and Neck Surgery at Henry Ford Hospital in Detroit, raced to the bedside of a woman who couldn't breathe. She had no idea that she was about to come face-to-face with a mysterious outbreak in patients who had recently undergone surgery.[282]

With more than two decades of experience under her belt, she had rescued countless patients who couldn't breathe from the brink of death. The causes ranged from major trauma in the aftermath of car wrecks, shootings, and strangulation to pneumonia, cancer, and severe allergic reactions. Yaremchuk was often called by her colleagues to perform tracheostomies, a surgical procedure in which she cuts a hole in a patient's windpipe and inserts a plastic tube that can be connected to a breathing machine.

When she arrived at the patient's bedside, the woman was in severe distress. She'd undergone cervical spine (neck) surgery several days earlier. In order to sort out the cause of the woman's respiratory distress, Yaremchuk asked to see the CAT scan of the patient's neck. She was unprepared for what she saw: "My first reaction was confusion. The patient had this massive inflammatory reaction in her neck. It wasn't an abscess or an infection. There wasn't anything that could explain the massive inflammation. It was something we'd never seen before—something that hadn't been described or talked about."

For Yaremchuk, the patient's presentation was so different, so new and unexpected, that she said, "It was like looking at the first AIDS patient."

She would soon get a clue to a possible cause of the woman's strange condition. As chair of the department of otorhinolaryngology, Yaremchuk is responsible for overseeing the training and work of resident doctors in the specialty commonly known as "ear, nose, and throat," or ENT. When she mentioned the woman's case to the young doctors, a few residents rolled their eyes and said they'd seen a couple of similar cases. One of them mentioned that neurosurgeons were implanting a new device during spine surgery that contained rhBMP-2 (recombinant bone morphogenetic protein 2), a biologic bone stimulator that is a component of a device known as Infuse. Yaremchuk wondered if this could be the cause of the problem. But she was circumspect: in medicine, mistaken associations are a dime a dozen. Yaremchuk says, "We were seeing something new, and I thought, 'Okay, as chair of the department, it's my responsibility to figure out what's going on.'"

As she puzzled through the problem, she says she realized there were two very unusual things about this spate of patients with respiratory distress. First was the fact that the distress was occurring at all, because there was nothing new about cervical spine surgery: these surgeries were common and had been done "for forever" without similar problems, she said. Second was that in the rare instances in which respiratory distress did occur in the past, it tended to be caused by bleeding that occurred either during surgery or in its immediate aftermath—not several days later and not caused by massive inflammation.

Yaremchuk dismissed the idea that a new neurosurgeon might be the source of the cases gone wrong. It seemed unlikely. These weren't botched surgeries, and a quick check showed that the patients with complications weren't treated by any one surgeon or group of surgeons.

Was it possible that rhBMP-2 was the culprit? She talked with some of the neurosurgeons. They assured her that rhBMP-2 was safe. Studies had shown it, and besides, it was in wide use.

But Yaremchuk wasn't convinced. Any single neurosurgeon might not be able to see the big picture, because he or she might not see enough patients to realize there's a problem, but Yaremchuk and her residents were seeing complications among the patients of all neurosurgeons in the large nine-hundred-bed teaching hospital. They were in a much better position to crack the case.

Determined to figure out whether rhBMP-2 was at the heart of the outbreak, she enlisted several colleagues to assist with a study. They compared the outcomes of all patients at Henry Ford Hospital who underwent cervical spine surgery with rhBMP-2 from 2004 to 2009 (260 patients) to those who underwent cervical spine surgery without rhBMP-2 (515 patients). The results were damning. Patients implanted with rhBMP-2 were more likely to develop problems, ranging from difficulty swallowing to respiratory distress and death. The numbers from her study suggested that 25 more patients per one thousand operations would die if rhBMP-2 was used during surgery.[283]

Other doctors began to see problems as well. One report in the MAUDE database stated that a patient developed "airway issues" and died two days after surgery.[284] Another report described a patient who experienced "difficulty swallowing, extreme pain, more pain after surgery, difficulty speaking, nerve injury, radiating pain to the legs...[and] bony overgrowth" and had to walk "hunched over." Yet another stated that a patient developed "acute respiratory failure" and died eight days after surgery. There were other reports. Many others. Invariably the maker of rhBMP-2 declared that it was only reporting the deaths "for notification purposes" and that it was "unable to determine the definitive cause of the reported event," because "neither the device nor films of applicable imaging studies were returned to the manufacturer."

After Yaremchuk published her study, three doctors sent a letter to the editor of the journal vigorously disputing her findings, saying that the data "completely contradict our experience."[285] Citing a study they published in 2010, the authors asserted that there were no deaths among the "more than 150 patients" they had followed for two years and that most problems were relatively minor and "self-limiting." Two of the three authors acknowledged that they received payments from Medtronic, Stryker, and other device manufacturers.

Nor was Medtronic about to take Yaremchuk's findings lying down. It, too, insisted that rhBMP-2 was safe and sent a letter to her demanding copies of the medical records of all the patients who were included in the study.

The bullying tactic didn't go over well with the hospital, and it refused to hand over the requested medical records. Hospital lawyers informed Medtronic that the company had no standing to request the personal records of patients.

The hospital's refusal to bow to industry demands may have been thanks in part to Yaremchuk herself. In January of 2007, as vice president of clinical practice performance, she helped to implement a systemwide "influence-free" policy.[286] The policy prohibits doctors from accepting gifts from drug or device manufacturers, including free drug samples, which are often used to influence doctors to prescribe expensive brand-name drugs. Doctors were banned from accepting even "pens, coffee mugs, or sticky notes from industry" (items that often come with the names of products emblazoned on them). Yaremchuk says that the policy was necessary because even though many doctors claim they aren't influenced by gifts, "every study shows that there is a subtle, but real, influence."

The Henry Ford Health System estimated in 2009 that it was saving $10 million per year in lower drug and device costs thanks to the policy prohibiting doctors from accepting gifts from industry.

When Yaremchuk helped to implement the influence-free policy, the Physician Payments Sunshine Act, which requires doctors to report money they receive from drug and device companies,[*] was still three years off in the future, and a wave of reforms aimed at transparency and limiting conflicts of interest was yet to follow. But her actions and those of others would lead to shocking revelations about Medtronic, the backstory about Infuse, the FDA, and extraordinary sums of money.

One of those revelations was that recombinant bone morphogenetic protein, rhBMP-2, had never been approved by the FDA for use in the neck—the most dangerous part of the spine for implantation. But that is a story best told by a Hollywood screenwriter, Jerome Lew.

---

[*] Under the act, the payments are posted publicly by the Centers for Medicare and Medicaid Services and by the investigative journalism outlet ProPublica, at https://projects.propublica.org/docdollars/.

* * *

To understand how surgeons came to implant rhBMP-2 in the cervical spine, it's necessary to follow a complex scheme carried out by industry. It's a story Jerome Lew would learn in excruciating detail after he had rhBMP-2 implanted in his neck. Lew has worked for directors of films such as *All the President's Men*, *Scarface*, and *Top Gun*, and he says what happened to him might be the subject of a horror film.

In February of 2009, Lew was bringing his newborn son home from the hospital—a day Lew would say "should have been joyous." But as he was taking his son out of the backseat, Lew was struck by a car. His son was unhurt, but Lew was injured. He was ultimately referred to Jeffrey C. Wang, then the chief of spine surgery at UCLA's Spine Center. After reviewing a CAT scan of Lew's cervical spine, Wang reportedly told him that he needed surgery or he could end up paralyzed.

A few months later, in May of 2009, still in profound pain, Lew underwent surgery, believing that he was about to have a routine neck fusion in which bits of bone taken from his hip would be used to fuse together vertebrae in his neck. By all accounts, the surgery appeared to be a success, and Lew says he had "dramatic" pain relief following the operation. But months later, the symptoms returned and worsened. He lost strength in his arms. He was clumsy when he tried to pick things up. The pain was unrelenting. Lew explained his symptoms to Wang, who suggested that he see a psychiatrist and a pain management specialist.

By 2012, things had gotten much worse. He was having trouble walking. His voice grew hoarse. Talking and swallowing foods became difficult. Eventually he began to lose bladder control, and at times he would urinate on himself.

Lew decided not to return to Wang. Instead he sought help from

Charles Rosen, a spine surgeon at the University of California, Irvine. When Rosen reviewed images of Lew's neck and his medical records, he found that Wang had implanted rhBMP-2 in Lew's neck and that it had triggered one of its dreaded complications—bony overgrowth. Bone was now impinging on nerves in Lew's neck.

Rosen undertook risky revision surgery on Lew, and although he was unable to remove the devices in Lew's neck, he was able to relieve some of the pressure on the nerves on one side of his spine, which gave Lew significant relief from his symptoms.

Recombinant bone morphogenetic protein was originally approved by the FDA in 2002 as part of a "combination product"—a biologic product and a mechanical device—known as Infuse. Manufactured by Medtronic, Infuse consists of special sponges that are impregnated with rhBMP-2 at the time of surgery and placed in a metal cage sized and shaped for the large bones of the lower spine. The FDA approved Infuse for use at only one disk level in the lower spine—not the neck.

Which brings us to the slippery issue of off-label use. Off-label use occurs when a drug or device that has been approved for one condition (as written on the product's label) is instead prescribed or implanted for a different use or condition. For example, an aspirin-like drug might be approved by the FDA to treat pain—but not to treat cancer. Doctors could *legally* prescribe an aspirinlike drug for cancer—an off-label use—but it's likely they would be held liable for harm to a patient if he or she died of an untreated cancer. On the other hand, many drugs, such as penicillin, have never been tested or approved for use in children, yet the use of penicillin to treat pneumonia in children is effective and widely used. Off-label prescribing carries certain risks and requires the physician to use judgment.

Complications of rhBMP-2 are generally related to two distinct problems. The first is an early, intense inflammatory reaction to the biologic product that occurs within several days of surgery. This is the type of reaction that first caught Yaremchuk's attention during the mysterious outbreak of respiratory distress at her institution. The second type of problem is a late-occurring complication caused by exuberant bony overgrowth, the complication that affected Lew. Bony overgrowth takes longer to develop and often occurs months after surgery. It can compress spinal nerves and the spinal cord itself, and impinge on structures in the neck, causing anything from difficulty breathing and swallowing to strokes, paralysis, and death.

While complications caused by rhBMP-2 in the lower spine (a use approved by the FDA) could include urinary incontinence and impotence, its complications when used off-label in the neck could be deadly because of its proximity to the airway and upper spine. Despite this, off-label use of rhBMP-2 was proving to be the rule, not the exception. One study found that between 85 and 96 percent of rhBMP-2 use is off-label.[287]

The dangers of implanting rhBMP-2 in the neck were known before Wang ever performed surgery on Lew. On July 1, 2008, more than nine months before Lew's operation, the FDA issued a warning about off-label use of rhBMP-2 in the neck, stating that it had received reports of "life-threatening complications" and that its "safety and effectiveness...in the cervical spine have not been demonstrated."[288] Unfortunately for many patients, implanting rhBMP-2 in the neck—an off-label use—would prove to be life-altering and life-threatening. Studies began to emerge showing that between a quarter and half of patients treated with Infuse and rhBMP-2 for on- and off-label uses would experience complications—including death.[289, 290] Some researchers reported a possible connection between rhBMP-2, which stimulates cell growth, and an increased risk of cancer activation or progression.[289, 291, 292]

Lew initiated legal proceedings against Wang, the surgeon who implanted BMP-2 in his neck. The tangled web of financial relationships, false claims by the manufacturers of spinal devices, and failed oversight by the FDA that he unearthed in the process explains a great deal about the dangers to patients inherent in the rise of the medical-industrial complex.

Lew charged in his suit that when Wang told him he needed surgery, he didn't disclose that he was a consultant for Medtronic and that he had research and financial ties to the company.[293] Together with two other spine-device manufacturers, Medtronic paid Wang $459,500 in speaker's fees and consultancies from 2004 to 2007. Wang also developed a technique for surgically implanting a plate manufactured by Biomet for which the company paid him $303,102 in royalties in 2011. It was the same plate Wang recommended for use at UCLA and that he implanted in Lew along with the Infuse component, rhBMP-2. And while Medtronic was funding Wang's research, Wang "consistently checked 'no'" on conflict-of-interest forms at UCLA when asked whether he received $500 or more from any company sponsoring his research.[295]

Wang wasn't the only UCLA faculty member who failed to declare his industry ties. According to Robert Pedowitz, the former chair of orthopedics at UCLA, the university benefited from turning a blind eye to financial conflicts.[296] Pedowitz charged in a whistleblower suit that industry payments to doctors and the university may have compromised patient care and that the university retaliated against him when he raised concerns, forcing him out of his position. In April of 2014, UCLA regents agreed to pay Pedowitz $10 million as part of a settlement agreement. In July of 2016, UCLA confirmed that it had also settled the case brought by Lew, for $4.2 million.[297] Medtronic separately entered into a confidential settlement with Lew.

The details of the story Lew brought to light in his lawsuit and in a presentation to the FDA can be difficult to follow. But the bottom line is this: Medtronic and other device companies promoted off-label use of rhBMP-2 by creating a spinal cage that was sized and shaped for the neck, allowing surgeons to implant rhBMP-2 in the neck and helping off-label use become the norm.

The FDA approved Infuse in 2002 as a high-risk class III device comprising a cage containing its component rhBMP-2, after going through the FDA's "most stringent" testing, or premarket approval (PMA) process. The device was used in the lower spine in clinical tests and was approved for that use only.

Soon after Infuse hit the market, the company manufactured a much smaller cage that fit into the small bones of the neck. Here's where things get tricky: by declaring that the new, smaller cage was intended for use in the *lower* spine and that it was "substantially equivalent" to the already approved cage used in that part of the body, the company was able to have the smaller cage, known as VERTE-STACK, cleared through the quickie, down-and-dirty 510(k) process, which doesn't require any clinical testing.

Because the VERTE-STACK cage is hollow, it can be used to implant rhBMP-2-impregnated sponges, which is exactly how surgeons began using it, because they knew its shape and size were right for the much smaller bones of the neck. It was a slick ruse: if Medtronic had openly stated that it wanted to sell the device for the neck, that would have constituted an entirely new use or indication and should have triggered a demand for clinical testing. But Medtronic sidestepped that hurdle (and expense) by saying that the tiny dime-sized cage was meant for the lower back.

So why didn't the FDA recognize the size difference and its implications when Medtronic submitted its 510(k) clearance application? The dimensions were clearly stated for anyone to see. Zafar Khan, a codeveloper of the cage, said he helped develop it specifically for use in the neck—a point that appears to have been either missed or glossed over by the FDA.[298]

Whether the FDA was rushed (the very problem the Institute of

Medicine said was causing serious problems at the agency), whether it was asleep at the wheel, or whether someone was in line for the revolving door between the FDA and industry is not clear, but the agency would fail again and again to protect the public despite multiple warnings from experts.

John W. Brantigan, an orthopedic surgeon who patented the first modern spinal cages, warned the FDA in 2003 that the agency was clearing spinal devices that were "impossible to use for the labeled purposes." In other words, a device labeled for use in the lower back but sized and shaped for the neck *couldn't possibly be used in the lower back*. Brantigan told the FDA that failing to require clinical trials of spinal cages would mean that "many patients will be subjected to unnecessary failures, chronic pain, and ruined lives."

His concerns were echoed by others.

Dr. Nancy E. Epstein, professor of clinical neurosurgery at the College of Medicine, State University of New York at Stony Brook and the chief of neurosurgical spine and education at NYU Winthrop-University Hospital, says she has seen serious problems with the use of rhBMP-2, especially when used off-label in the neck.[299] She and a colleague conducted a one-year study (2010) at one institution and found that complications were common. They found that 96 percent (170 of 177) of patients were treated off-label at a cost of $4,547,822; and of those treated off-label, nearly one in five patients (18.8 percent) underwent reoperation within just one year.[287]

Epstein conducted a separate review of 183 patients who had been offered operations by spine surgeons, and she determined that many didn't need surgery at all.[300]

But even before Yaremchuk and Epstein reported their findings, there had been warning signs that something was wrong with Medtronic research.

Eugene J. Carragee, professor of orthopedic surgery at Stanford

University and editor in chief of *The Spine Journal,* began to hear about "frequent and occasionally catastrophic complications" associated with rhBMP-2 and Infuse. Yet industry-sponsored research reported virtually no serious complications. Carragee was suspicious. He said, "Their results were simply too good. Medtronic said thirteen published RCTs [randomized controlled trials] involving eight-hundred-plus patients showed there were no 'BMP-2 related' complications despite using the potent growth factor at approximately one million times the normal concentration" in humans.[301]

As an editor, Carragee knew plenty about scientific literature becoming distorted when industry-supported authors downplay harms of medical devices and drugs by submitting only positive results for publication. And he knew something about conflicts of interest. The sums the authors were raking in from Medtronic were simply stupendous. "It was more money than anything we'd seen before," he said, citing payments of more than $23 million paid to one author and $6 million paid to a handful of doctors who coauthored articles about the device while failing to mention the known dangers.[302] A 2013 Senate investigation would find that Medtronic paid a total of approximately $210 million to physician authors who failed to report adverse events.[303] And doctors were paid kickbacks to implant the device: one consulting agreement showed that spine doctors would be paid $4,000 a day for "services performed."[304]

Determined to understand the divergent claims about the safety of the device, Carragee and his colleagues at Stanford launched their own study. They analyzed safety and efficacy data reported in the thirteen original industry-sponsored studies, then compared those results with data they obtained from the FDA. *The Spine Journal* published the results in 2011: at a minimum, with greater than 99 percent statistical confidence, the risk of harms associated with

Infuse were ten to fifty times higher than what was stated in the Medtronic-sponsored peer-reviewed publications.[290]

For his efforts, Carragee was rewarded in 2013 with a two-year barrage of attacks led by the device entrepreneur and industry consultant Robin R. Young, who sought to have Carragee removed as editor of *The Spine Journal.* Young, who is not a physician, charged that Carragee was failing readers of the journal because "he has abandoned even the pretense of impartiality," and he alleged that Carragee "accuses researchers of financial bias where none, in fact exists." Young had a pulpit from which to preach: he is also the publisher of *Orthopedics This Week,* an industry publication, and in it, he published his editorial under the headline CARRAGEE MUST RESIGN, written in all-capital letters and set in a massive font.[305]

But Carragee, a former lieutenant colonel in the Army Reserve Medical Corps who was seriously wounded in Iraq, is not someone to blink under fire. His research on the device had been vetted by peer reviewers, including the dean of Stanford's medical school. Carragee says, "I was a tenured professor at Stanford, and I wasn't worried about my job." Instead he was worried that patients were being harmed and that his profession was being sullied by what he called "Elmer Gantry–style revival meetings" where rhBMP-2 and Infuse were promoted by individuals on Medtronic's payroll, writing, "Ten years after BMP-2's introduction, we cannot identify a single well-proven area of benefit, but we know it can kill you in the cervical spine and probably can promote cancer, which can then kill you."[305]

Despite reports of adverse events long known to the company, Medtronic was not to be deterred. Even though off-label use of Infuse was increasingly common, Medtronic anticipated even more sales if it could legally and openly promote the device for use in the neck. The company was upbeat about the possibilities and told its shareholders that Infuse would become the "standard of care in spinal fusion therapy."[306]

To win the right to legally promote additional uses, the company would have to first submit a study to the FDA showing that the device was safe and effective for each additional use. The company did undertake a study—however, the results were disastrous. But rather than report the bad outcomes, it kept mum.

The whole matter only came to light more than a decade later, when three investigative reporters with the Minneapolis *Star Tribune* published a report in April of 2016 entitled "Question of Risk: Medtronic's Lost Study."[306] As in the case of the VNS and other devices, the MAUDE database reflected only a small part of the problem. More than a thousand injuries and deaths associated with rhBMP-2 from 2002 to 2007 had been dubbed commercial trade secrets and were not made public.[229, 306]

The study had little (if any) scientific merit, though Medtronic said it employed the study design after consulting with someone at the FDA, but it declined to tell the *Star Tribune* who that someone was. The company had obtained the data by asking doctors for reports on roughly one out of every ten patients implanted with Infuse. After collecting reports on 3,600 patients, it had uncovered more than one thousand injuries and a handful of deaths. This was not good news for Medtronic. And it wasn't likely to win a new approval from the FDA. Rather than present the entire data set, Medtronic presented a small subset of selected cases to the FDA, requesting broader approval for use. The FDA turned Medtronic down.[306]

By 2011, several state attorneys general and the Senate finance committee had gotten wind of problems with the device and subpoenaed documents from Medtronic, requesting information on all associated adverse events. According to the *Star Tribune* reporters, "Medtronic handed over thousands of pages—but not the retrospective study, which the company says was misfiled in its archives."

The company shut down the study in the spring of 2008. At

that time, there were only 261 adverse events reported in the FDA's database. More than five years after the study was ended and long after the thirty-day reporting requirement was over, Medtronic approached the FDA about how to report the 1,024 adverse events it had collected years earlier. The FDA took no action against Medtronic for late reporting, even though the agency had previously sent warning letters in 2009 and 2011 to the company for failure to report adverse events. When the FDA released a three-sentence summary of the study in 2013, it blacked out the number of adverse events, redacted on behalf of Medtronic as a "corporate trade secret,"[306] only releasing the total number after the *Star Tribune* criticized the agency's suppression of important information.

★ ★ ★

Even industry insiders, who should be the most knowledgeable consumers of healthcare, can be victimized by the careless use of devices for off-label purposes.

Medtronic executive Kimberly Pickett started out as a sales representative at the company in 2005. She had been pre-med, has an outgoing personality, and is attractive—a combination prized by companies that use representatives to sell devices to doctors. Representatives are given expense accounts and encouraged to schmooze doctors. They take them out for meals, tell them about their companies' products, set up educational meetings, and cultivate doctors they designate as key opinion leaders (KOLs).

Pickett started out in the gastrointestinal division of Medtronic, but by 2007 she had moved over to the prestigious cardiovascular group, where she would specialize in artificial heart valves and other implanted cardiovascular devices. When she began her training, she says, "I got about twelve binders dropped at my front door." The huge binders from Medtronic contained vast amounts of data and information. She was expected to learn every aspect of cardiac anatomy and function as well as the pressure gradients within the heart and the great vessels. She also had to learn every detail about the devices she would sell: what conditions they treated, how they were constructed, which FDA regulations governed each device, and which surgical approaches were right for each device.

Pickett loved her job. She had a strong anatomy background from her years in pre-med, and those twelve fat binders were just one part of a bigger challenge she thrived on. The company sent her to a lab to perform valve surgery on dead pig hearts—and, once, on a live pig. She recalls, "That one was hard for me because I'm an animal lover, but they treated the pigs very humanely. . . . As far as I know, he [the pig] is still alive today."

Because surgeons often deal with devices from several companies, and because each device can require a different approach, surgeons often want a manufacturer's representative in the OR with them. Eventually Pickett was flying across the country and spending up to four or five hours per case in operating rooms at the "head of the table" with cardiothoracic surgeons as she guided them through the details of implanting Medtronic's artificial heart valves.

Pickett was a hard worker and was good at what she did. So good that she rose through the ranks with surprising speed. By the time she was thirty-seven, she had been promoted to an executive position as Medtronic's director of strategic sales for the cardiac and vascular group. She was responsible for multimillion-dollar accounts with hospitals in California and Arizona. Her salary and compensation package put her income on par with that of a typical cardiologist.

Not only was she thriving in her profession, she also truly believed in what she was doing. Medtronic's heart valves were FDA-approved and had extensive long-term data to support their safety and efficacy. No question that those heart valves saved lives.

Pickett was also a company loyalist. Once, she participated in a go-kart race at a company team-building event during which a colleague tried to pass her and snagged her rear wheel, causing her vehicle to slam into the racetrack wall. It was a hard impact, and her head snapped back, causing immediate pain in her neck. Despite her pain, she returned to work right away. She was not one to take sick time. Nor did she want to make waves, so she didn't ask her manager to file an incident report, which was required but which he neglected to do.

The initial pain of the injury, instead of subsiding, as she had hoped, began to get worse. Severe nerve pain began shooting from her neck down her left arm and into her hand and fingers, which became completely numb. She saw a doctor who said she would need surgery. Pickett held off. She sought second, third, and fourth opinions, hoping the pain would just go away—or that she'd find a doctor who would tell her she didn't need surgery. But every doctor told her the same thing: there was no way around surgery. After months of pain and sleepless nights, she finally turned to her colleagues in the Medtronic spine division for help and asked for the name of the best spine surgeons between Arizona and California.

A colleague gave her three names: Jeffrey Wang,[*] Rick Delamarter, and Todd Lanman. She saw Lanman, a Beverly Hills neurosurgeon and doctor to the stars (his office boasts pictures of Clint Eastwood, Liza Minnelli, and Sylvester Stallone). Lanman told her she would need "four levels" of repair—two artificial disks and two fusions.

Pickett says, "He showed me a couple of the [artificial] disks and said, 'I'll use a Medtronic and a Synthes [product].' He mentioned Infuse. I had no idea what Infuse was. I'd never even heard the

---

[*] Wang is the surgeon who operated on Jerome Lew.

word before. He told me that he 'may or may not' use it." She says when she asked what Infuse was, Lanman told her only that it 'helps solidify the fusion.'" Pickett says she's not one to hang back: she asks a lot of questions because, as she says, "I know too much." She asked Lanman if there was anything she should be concerned about. His response, she says, was "laid back" and "reassuring."

But Pickett knew that all surgeries carry a certain degree of risk. She told Lanman she wanted two things. She wanted her surgery to be performed at Cedars-Sinai, a hospital where she had corporate accounts and whose processes, which she described as excellent, she had come to trust. She also wanted her surgery done first thing on a Monday morning, when the OR was at its cleanest and the staff at its sharpest.

According to her legal complaint filed against Lanman and Medtronic,[*] Lanman, who had privileges at Cedars-Sinai, nonetheless told Pickett he preferred to do the surgery at Olympia Medical Center, which he referred to as a "boutique hospital," because he had his own staff there. Pickett acquiesced.

The night before the surgery, Lanman's office faxed Pickett a written consent form. "It was a consent form for carte blanche," says Pickett. "It said he might use a variety of different devices, bioabsorbables, BMP—and I didn't even know that BMP was Infuse, because that wasn't the word he'd used." She was alarmed by the list of potential complications: along with infection and bleeding were paralysis, stroke, and death. Pickett says she called Lanman's office and told the staff, "'I'm not signing this.' But they told me, 'Well, you have to sign it or you have to cancel the surgery.' I asked to talk to Lanman, but they said he was in Hawaii and wouldn't get in until

---

[*] *Kimberly Pickett v. Todd H. Lanman, M.D., Inc; Olympia Medical Center; Medtronic, Inc., Medtronic Sofamor Danek USA, Inc., and DOES 2-100.* Filed December 10, 2013. Lanman has denied the charges in Pickett's complaint.

the morning right before my surgery. I told them I still wanted to talk with him before I'd agree to surgery."

The next morning, on June 25, 2012, she got to the hospital at seven. Pickett says Lanman came to see her just before 1:30 p.m. "He came in all cocky talking about his surfing trip. I said, 'Hey, we need to talk about this consent form—it's ridiculous,' and he said, 'Hey, kiddo, you have to sign this. You know how it goes: you have to sign stuff like this.'" He added, "You have nothing to worry about." Exhausted, Pickett yielded. She says she felt bullied into signing the waiver.

"What happened next," says Pickett, "changed my life forever."

According to her complaint, Lanman implanted rhBMP-2 in Pickett's neck. Several days after surgery, Pickett developed an intense inflammatory reaction that paralyzed her vocal cords. Doctors repeatedly injected steroids and fillers directly into her vocal cords in an attempt to allow her to recover her ability to speak normally. It was a scary time, because if the swelling didn't go down, she could have trouble breathing, a complication that has forced some implanted patients to go on life support and even die.[289, 307]

Eventually she did recover from the inflammatory reaction, and though the numbness in her arm persisted, the pain began to let up. She returned to work full-time and continued to enjoy unusual success.

Then, five to six months after surgery, the nerve pain returned with a vengeance, affecting both sides of her neck. The pain in her left arm was "excruciating." By this time, Pickett had done some reading and learned that BMP-2 can trigger ectopic, or excess, bone growth. She asked Lanman if that could be the problem, but he said no, that he'd just "missed a spot," implying that the problem was caused by her underlying injury—not the device he'd implanted. Besides, he added, the claim about bony overgrowth was just some hype caused by overzealous attorneys trying to make money.

She sought second and third opinions from doctors who read the scans and told her that the cause of her pain was crystal clear: rhBMP-2 had indeed caused significant bony overgrowth and was impinging on her nerves. The excess bone would have to be carefully drilled away.

In May of 2013, she underwent revision surgery, this time by a surgeon in her home state of Arizona. When he opened her up, he described what he saw as a "shit show." The bone was wrapped around her spine and nerves. He had to use exquisite care as he drilled away at the excess bone. Nonetheless, one of her vertebrae fractured as he attempted to free her nerves from the mass of excess bone.

By that time she had asked her boss to file an incident report regarding the accident at the team-building event. If nothing else, she wanted to file for worker's compensation to help pay for her medical expenses (even though she'd continued to work full-time, she was paying extensive medical bills out of pocket and with her private health insurance), and she needed the incident report to show that her injury was work-related. She also asked for medical articles about complications related to the device. But, she says, Medtronic dismissed her concerns, saying that "hungry attorneys" were creating unnecessary panic. If she wanted medical articles, she'd have to get them from her surgeon. She scoffs, "Clearly that wasn't going to happen."

She told her boss she had to undergo a second surgery because of bony overgrowth caused by rhBMP-2, and she thought an adverse event report should be filed with Medtronic's Office of Medical Affairs. But he demurred. So Pickett went to Medtronic's Tempe, Arizona, office and filed an adverse event report herself.

Suddenly, despite her continued excellent work ratings, Medtronic informed her that her position was being eliminated. She was out of a job.

After two operations, out of work, in pain, and facing the possibility of even more surgery, she finally decided to file suit against the company she loved. In the process, she, like Lew before her, would learn a good deal about the device implanted in her neck—and the stupendous sums of money involved.

One of the first things she learned about was the FDA warning issued in 2008, four years before her surgery, notifying healthcare providers that rhBMP-2 used in the cervical spine was associated with "life-threatening complications."[288] The agency urged practitioners to "either use approved alternative treatments or consider enrolling as investigators in approved clinical studies."

Why hadn't Lanman told her of this warning?

Then, according to her complaint, she learned something else about Lanman: he was a prominent consultant for Medtronic, which had paid him more than $1 million in fees and royalties. Not only had he failed to tell her about the lavish payments he received from Medtronic, he also didn't tell her the reason he may not have wanted to do the surgery at Cedars-Sinai: he *couldn't* do the surgery there, because the hospital had significant restrictions on the off-label use of rhBMP-2 due to its known harmful effects. But, according to Pickett, in her complaint, Lanman's "boutique" hospital, Olympia, had no such prohibition.

Pickett says that when she asked her Medtronic colleague who specialized in spine devices about Infuse, he didn't tell her its use in the neck would be off-label. "The only thing he said was, 'It's great stuff.'" She says she never would have agreed to be implanted with rhBMP-2 if she had been told about the dangers of its off-label use. She says Medtronic's official position is that representatives shouldn't promote off-label use: "We're told to walk out of the room if a doctor uses a device off-label." She says they played it by the book "one hundred percent" in the cardiovascular section.

Nonetheless, off-label sales are the bread and butter of orthopedic surgeons using rhBMP-2, and some of the largest users of rhBMP-2 are surgeons with ties to Medtronic.[287, 296, 297]

How did off-label use of rhBMP-2 come to be such a common practice among surgeons if manufacturers are prohibited from promoting devices and drugs for off-label use?

Sales representatives are quick to say that there is often an implicit "wink-wink, nod-nod" attitude about off-label promotion—a strategy that ensures a financial boon for both the company and its reps. Sales reps say the pressure to meet sales quotas is enormous—so enormous that it can, and does, lead to the use of widespread illicit tactics by companies and reps.

Former Cyberonics representative Andrew J. Hagerty, joined by the US government, charged in a whistle-blower lawsuit against Cyberonics that bosses at the company set sales quotas for the VNS device that its reps could only have met by participating in illicit promotions.[308, 309] According to the complaint, if reps failed to meet 75 percent of a revenue goal in a single quarter, they would be put under a special supervisory plan, and if they didn't fully meet their quotas the following quarter, they were terminated. But companies typically employ both carrots and sticks, and the complaint stated that "almost one-third of sales representatives earned more than $360,000 per year with more than 66 percent of that amount coming from commissions."

The combination of potentially fantastic earnings and the constant threat of being fired for "underperforming" can lead representatives to engage in unethical and fraudulent practices. When one top-performing rep was found to have created her own marketing materials, which hadn't been approved by the company (and therefore may have violated the FDA's approved labeling of the VNS device), Cyberonics didn't fire her, nor did it take away her high-earner commissions. Instead it simply withheld an all-expenses-paid trip to her choice of Alaska, Hawaii, Tahiti, or the Bahamas. In this way, representatives—like their companies—learn that paying certain penalties is merely the cost of doing business.

Companies and their reps beef up sales by cultivating doctors through a combination of flattery and "consulting," or speaker's, fees, and Hagerty's suit exposed the multilayered conflicts of interest that connect industry and doctors in the promotion of off-label prescribing and outright fraud.

Pickett hopes that her suit will create awareness of the fact that patients need to ask a lot of questions. She says, "Don't assume your doctor is making the best decision for you. Some may make the decision best for their pocket."

One doctor who has an intimate understanding of industry influence is Daniel Carlat, associate clinical professor of psychiatry at Tufts University School of Medicine. Carlat was flattered when a Wyeth drug representative asked him in 2001 to give talks to other doctors about its antidepressant drug venlafaxine (marketed in the US as Effexor XR). He'd be paid $500 for a one-hour talk over a free lunch—$750 if he had to drive for an hour to get there.[310, 311]

Carlat, who specializes in psychopharmacology, says he didn't believe at first that he was doing anything wrong when he agreed to give the talks. He was familiar with studies showing that the drug might be more effective than some older antidepressants. Since he had already prescribed the drug to a few patients with some success, he reasoned that he would be doing nothing unethical by talking about the drug's benefits.

The company flew Carlat and his wife to a "faculty development" program in New York City, where they were put up for two nights at a luxury hotel and given tickets to a Broadway show. Carlat quickly discovered that some of the biggest names in psychiatry were also attending—and benefiting from Wyeth's largesse. It was a heady experience. While there, Carlat ran into an old colleague who mentioned that he was giving talks promoting gabapentin

(Neurontin) for Warner Lambert—a drug he said was "great" for some patients with bipolar disorder. Carlat was surprised by his old friend's claim because of his own experience of prescribing the drug and because a study of gabapentin prescribed for bipolar disorder showed that the drug failed to perform better than a placebo. In a comedic moment, Carlat, seemingly oblivious to the process he himself was undergoing, wondered whether his colleague's "positive opinion had been influenced by the money he was paid to give talks."

After attending the faculty development program, for which he received an honorarium, Carlat was off and running, teaching doctors about venlafaxine. Over time, however, Carlat learned about some problems with the drug and decided to give more balanced presentations. At the very next talk, when he was open about the limited efficacy and side effects of the drug, Wyeth representatives took note. A corporate district manager was dispatched to follow up with Carlat and let him know that the company was aware that his most recent presentation was less "enthusiastic" than usual. Then, in a moment that would prove to be the grenade under Carlat's feet, the manager asked Carlat, solicitously, "Have you been sick?" It was Carlat's moment of truth.

Carlat wasn't sick. Although he says it's possible that the district manager's question about his health was a genuine expression of concern, it was this question—and its timing—that brought everything into focus for him. It made him realize, as he later said, "something I would never, never have predicted happened: I ended up being a cog in their marketing machine."

Carlat immediately resigned as a speaker for Wyeth and decided that the best way to atone for the inflated picture he'd painted about venlafaxine and the $30,000 he had received for giving talks over the previous year was to go on a "march of shame" in which he would give free "undrug talks" to any group that asked him to. By "coming clean" with his story, Carlat said, "I'm hoping to convince doctors to give up their addiction to industry money. Ultimately, our professionalism is at stake. We want our men and women to come in from the dark side."

Fortunately he didn't try to put a pretty face on his own behavior. In his own account, published in the *New York Times,* he described how drug companies bring doctors into the world of industry-sponsored "medical education"—and how doctors may embark on such relationships without any intent of harm or deceit but can nevertheless be slowly seduced into questionable behaviors, such as making pumped-up claims of drugs' effectiveness while failing to give full weight to their side effects. In the article, Carlat presents his conduct warts and all, and you can almost smell his sweat as he quivers before a fellow doctor who, he fears, sees him for what he is: "a drug rep with an MD" degree.

In January of 2003, he launched the *Carlat Psychiatry Report.* Its website states, "We receive no corporate funding, which allows a clear-eyed evaluation of all available treatments."

Each player in the dramas that Lew, Pickett, and Carlat were caught up in, including the surgeons, the hospitals, the manufacturers, and manufacturers' representatives, stood to benefit financially by promoting the companies' respective products and by obscuring their very real dangers. There is no conspiracy in any of this—just a confluence of interests that stretches across the entire healthcare industry.

Chapter Eleven

BREAKDOWN

DENNIS FEGAN REMAINED CONVINCED that the VNS "cure" caused his asystole—and probably the deaths of many less fortunate individuals. He wanted the FDA to pay attention. And if it wouldn't, he'd make sure the world knew.

Fegan sent an e-mail query to the FDA asking why seizures weren't listed as a potential side effect of the VNS device. On April 24, 2009, he received an e-mail he wasn't supposed to see. Ann Costello, the FDA reviewer who had served on the panel to approve the VNS device, accidentally responded to an e-mail thread started by Fegan's inquiry by clicking "reply all." It was a hasty click, and she must have instantly regretted it. The discussions that followed Fegan's original e-mail were supposed to be internal FDA deliberations. Costello immediately put out a recall on the e-mail, but it was too late. Within seconds, Fegan had the draft version of the FDA's response, along with suggested edits. The original, unedited message read:

Dear Mr. Fegan,

This is what I have heard from our Office of Device Evaluation:

The most current approved labeling listed with FDA has potential for increased seizures...and it is as a side effect. It was in the original labeling, removed and was subsequently told to be put back in. Approved per supplement 63."

Thank You,
Joseph Tartal, Technical Branch Chief

In response to Tartal's draft version, Costello wrote:

"I would delete the statement 'It was in the original labeling, removed and was subsequently told to be put back in. Approved per supplement 63' as this is not public knowledge."

Not public knowledge? Whom was the FDA protecting? Itself? Cyberonics? Had the agency granted permission to the company to remove seizures as a listed side effect? The information was put back in the company's manuals in December of 2008, but it was not to be found in an earlier version.

Costello's e-mail made one thing clear: the FDA seemed more concerned with protecting Cyberonics and itself than with protecting the public interest.

With the FDA ignoring him, Fegan was determined to get his story out to the press. By late 2010, my colleague, Shannon Brownlee, and I had written three articles about the device industry in which Fegan's case appeared, including my original article in *The BMJ* and two popular articles in *Discover* and *Reader's Digest*.[100, 312, 313] They included what I thought was one of the most shocking points of the case: Cyberonics never collected death statistics for any of the five studies the company submitted to the FDA to prove the safety of the VNS device. And even more shocking to me: the FDA said it was satisfied that the device was safe based on the studies provided by Cyberonics.

Fegan sent the articles out to everyone he could think of. More politicians. More journalists. More FDA officials. He struggled to get the word out for more than a year after the articles about the VNS device were published. But by 2012, it was clear that the articles had changed absolutely nothing. There was no public outcry. No calls for a congressional investigation. No action taken at the FDA.

In August of 2012, Fegan wrote to Dr. Jeffrey E. Shuren, the director of the Center for Drug Evaluation and Research, a division of the FDA:

Dear Dr. Shuren,

I would like share my near death experience with you. On July 2 2006, I had what I thought was a bad run of atonic seizures. My parents just happened to stop by that Sunday morning and realized something was terribly wrong with me. They called my neurologist and EMS.

My last memory of that morning was being inside of the ambulance the next thing I knew I was in the ICU.

The Vagus Nerve Stimulator was stopping my heart (asystole) every 3 minutes during the 30 second stimulation cycles. If my parents hadn't happened to stop by that day I would have died and my death would have probably just been written off as a fatal seizure or SUDEP. No one would have ever suspected it was the VNS that killed me. . . .

Dennis Fegan

But none of his entreaties was met with any action. Still, Fegan had one last spark of hope. One of the officials Fegan had contacted was William H. Maisel, deputy director for science and chief scientist at the FDA's Center for Devices and Radiological Health. A cardiologist and an assistant professor of medicine at Harvard Medical School, Maisel had long been a strong advocate for improved safety standards for implanted medical devices. He founded the Medical Device Safety Institute before he moved to the FDA. Maisel had responded to Fegan personally and promised that he would oversee an investigation into the VNS device.[314]

Then, suddenly, Maisel stopped responding.

Fegan was now in free fall. He was sure the device was still killing people with epilepsy—people no one seemed to care about. He felt as if he were screaming, yet the world had gone deaf. His thoughts were getting scary. He began to see signs that the Secret Service was on his doorstep in retaliation for his making threats against the FDA. The CIA was after him, too.

On September 11, 2012, Fegan sent a volley of e-mails to Maisel. He demanded that the agency remove all VNS devices from the market. When he didn't get an immediate response, he exploded:

> *Do you know who I am Bill? . . . Order every one of those GODDAMN VNS devices shut off NOW. Don't FUCK AROUND. Order every one of those GODDAMN devices off right this FUCKING minute before it kills one more innocent epileptic. If it doesn't happen NOW you will not only be having the law to deal with, your poor ass will have to deal with me.*
>
> *NOW GODDAMN IT.*
>
> *Dennis Fegan*

Maisel's failure to respond to Fegan may have been related to an incident two months earlier, in late July, when Maisel was arrested in a sting operation for soliciting a prostitute.[315] FDA leadership declined to take action against Maisel, saying that the arrest had nothing to do with his work at the FDA. Under the circumstances, Maisel, previously outspoken about device safety, wasn't sticking his head above the parapet. He was lucky to have a job.

Frustrated, Fegan sent other e-mails, equally threatening and equally out of character for him—at least for the old Dennis Fegan, whom his friends and family had always known.

Two days after sending his e-mails to Maisel, Fegan was whisked off to the psych ward at the Corpus Christi Medical Center. Neighbors had called the police because he was yelling and throwing lawn chairs in the street. When the police arrived, he told them he was building a barricade. Preparing for war. The CIA or the FDA, maybe both, were after him. He calmed down after a day or two at the Corpus Christi hospital and returned to what seemed a normal life.

But less than a year later, Fegan's big breakdown occurred.

Officer Ernesto Coronado was one of the first police officers to arrive at the home of Fegan's parents on August 25, 2013. Fegan and his sister were standing in front of the house when Coronado arrived. Fegan was obviously angry, and his movements appeared erratic. The officers tried to calm him and figure out what was upsetting him, but he was having none of it. Faced with an angry six-foot-three-inch, 240-pound man, Coronado and his colleague called for backup. Within minutes, two additional officers arrived. Four police cars were then parked in front of the house, their blue and red lights whirling, attracting the attention of neighbors.

At one point, Fegan threw a bottle, and it shattered on the sidewalk. At another point, he grabbed his sister's neck from behind. Fegan would later say it was "just a hug."

Unable to calm Fegan, one of the officers gave a small, almost imperceptible hand signal, and all four cops leaped into action. As Coronado would later write in his report, the officers "escorted [Fegan] to the ground."[316] Coronado was cut as he fell on shards of broken glass from the bottle Fegan had thrown. Still bleeding, Coronado and the other officers hog-tied Fegan. They put him face-down on the ground, bending his knees so his feet pointed up in the air. They cuffed his ankles and tied his ankle cuffs to his wrists, which were also cuffed behind his back. Then they dragged him off to one of the police vehicles. Fegan yelled and struggled as they put him in the car belly down across the backseat.

When police brought Fegan back to the psychiatric ward of the Corpus Christi hospital, Carlos Estrada, a psychiatrist, marked the admitting complaint with a description of Fegan as exhibiting "strange behavior." He wrote, "The patient is a 54-year-old white, single disabled male, who lives alone in Corpus Christi, Texas...the patient reports that he suffers from severe, uncontrolled temporal lobe epilepsy."

Estrada outlined what Fegan told him: that he had a VNS device implanted in 2000 that caused him to pass out when his heart stopped and that he had "started to investigate if the device was safe" by contacting Cyberonics as well as the FDA and other patients through the VNS message board. Fegan told Estrada that the device caused many deaths, and he wanted the device removed from the market. He said he couldn't sue the company for the harm he suffered because the Supreme Court ruled that as long as the FDA approved the device, the manufacturer was immune from lawsuits.

The psychiatrist faithfully noted each of Fegan's statements in his chart, revealing that Fegan was surprisingly lucid.

Estrada said that, while in the psychiatric unit, Fegan started "calling, writing, and e-mailing" FDA officials William Maisel and Jeffrey Shuren and that Fegan had become "obsessed" with the issue. Based on information provided by Fegan, his family, and one of Fegan's e-mails, Estrada wrote that Fegan was frustrated with the lack of action at the FDA and "made threatening e-mails using coarse language." Estrada quoted one of Fegan's e-mails (delicately changing "fuck" to "f***" in his notes): 'I don't see any signs of action yet...so get your f***ing ass in gear. I am not f***ng around here. You don't know me and you sure as f**k don't want to know me...'"

Fegan told Estrada that Homeland Security contacted him after his last e-mail, on September 11, 2012, and told him he was "going to be receiving a letter to 'cease and desist,' otherwise he would be prosecuted by the Federal Government."

Fegan rapidly improved during his stay in the psychiatric unit and was released from the hospital four days later, coherent and normal. But the episode left its mark. He felt humiliated, like a man who had tumbled far from the days when he was a professional paramedic calming and treating patients in crisis. Somehow his life seemed to have gone terribly, terribly wrong. He wasn't that violent, out-of-control man who'd been dragged from his parents' lawn by police.

These two episodes represented the first times Fegan had ever needed psychiatric care. He'd never been on psychiatric medication or had psychiatric problems in the past, yet he had suffered psychosis, a distinct condition in which an individual can't distinguish reality from unreality. Psychosis is a feature of schizophrenia, which causes some patients to hallucinate and see or hear things that don't exist. Schizophrenia usually begins early in life, typically in a patient's late teens or early twenties. A psychotic episode that begins late in life (Fegan was fifty-four) suggests a medical or organic problem rather than a psychiatric disorder. Metabolic disorders, toxic illnesses, severe infections involving the bloodstream or brain, dementia, and Alzheimer's disease are just a few of the medical problems that can cause psychoses. But Fegan wasn't demented or seriously ill. In between the two episodes he was normal. Nor was he schizophrenic.

There were reasons to suspect an organic basis for his breaks with reality. When he was hospitalized with multiple episodes of asystole, his brain was deprived of oxygen—a condition called hypoxia—which could have caused some injury to the brain. Larry Johnson, the ER doctor who cared for Fegan, said, "It wouldn't be surprising if he did have some degree of hypoxic brain damage."

Repeated episodes of oxygen deprivation may have set up Fegan for his unraveling those many years later, even though he was lucid in between, because stressors sometimes "unmask" underlying disorders. There are many parallels in medicine. For example, if someone has a so-called lytic lesion, an eaten-out area of bone caused by a cyst or cancer, he or she might walk around for years without any awareness of the problem—until a very slight trauma occurs and the bone shatters, unmasking the underlying cancer. So although Fegan's first psychotic break didn't occur until years after he was hospitalized with asystole, it could be that aggravating factors had unmasked underlying insults to his brain. And Fegan suffered a thousand small cuts—and several big ones—after he was hospitalized. Underlying hypoxic brain injury, combined with his original head injury at the age of seven, his temporal lobe seizures and seizure medicines, the chronic stress of his battle over the VNS device, and, finally, the ultimate and crushing blow of the Supreme Court ruling may have formed the substrate for Fegan's eruption.

For Fegan, it was as if he'd been fighting his way out of a thick tangle of spiderwebs, and the more he fought and struggled, the more entangled and hopeless he became. When he opened the letter from attorney Jay Winckler telling him that he couldn't sue Cyberonics because of the US Supreme Court ruling on preemption,[317] Fegan had already felt the earth shift beneath his feet. A Reagan-loving Texan, he believed in freewheeling capitalist enterprise, unfettered by government constraints. But the same lack of constraints on business, when applied to the healthcare industry, had caused him to live with a dangerous medical device in his neck, one that couldn't (and can't) be removed. Fegan's experiences upended some of his earlier beliefs. He still distrusts government, but he can also imagine it as a potential force for good—one that can provide genuine protections for citizens if it can be disentangled from the powerful arm of industry.

For Fegan, the medical-industrial complex isn't an abstraction. It's Cyberonics; it's the FDA; it's hospitals, doctors, insurers, medical researchers—and all of these failed him.

* * *

One final story from Fegan's medical history sums up in a small, sad way just how dysfunctional our American healthcare system can be.

Back in 2006, during Fegan's hospitalization, an X-ray had suggested that the lead wire from his VNS device appeared to have migrated dangerously into his jugular vein. Fegan was told of the finding but was reassured by his doctors that it was just a mistake— the lead was not in his jugular vein. Years later, his new neurologist, JoAnne Sullivan, decided to get a definitive reading on the VNS lead wire and ordered an ultrasound. The new test, performed on January 10, 2011, confirmed the original reading: the wire was indeed inside Fegan's jugular vein. The finding was so worrying that the radiologist, Cameron Gates, took the unusual step of contacting Sullivan by phone about the result and documenting in his note that: "The above findings and impression were discussed with [Sullivan] at 11:00 a.m. on 1/10/11. She expressed understanding of the findings during our conversation." Radiologists may read hundreds of imaging studies in a week. The overwhelming majority never trigger a phone call. But, said Gates, radiologists are required to call the referring doctor for potentially life- or limb-threatening circumstances in which further action or diagnostic testing must be taken to avert possible catastrophe. However, rather than alerting Fegan to a problem and calling in a specialist to evaluate him further, Sullivan simply ordered a repeat ultrasound—five months later, in June of 2011. This time a different radiologist confirmed the earlier finding. Once again, Sullivan failed to inform Fegan and instead ordered a *third* ultrasound, which was performed in October and which resulted in yet another radiologist reporting exactly the same finding that the three previous radiologists had reported: the VNS wire was in fact in Fegan's left jugular vein.

Fegan says that during an office visit with Sullivan, he noticed that she looked worried while she read one of the reports. He asked if something was wrong. She told him that the report indicated that the lead wires "weren't where they should be," he said, but that it was simply a "logical mistake" because of all the scarring in the area. Fegan says she reassured him that the leads were on the vagus nerve.

With Fegan's permission, in late 2015, fifteen years after he was implanted with the VNS device, I sent copies of his ultrasounds to Stephen Baker, a nationally recognized radiologist, and asked him to comment on the location of the leads. Baker became the fifth doctor to confirm that not only was the wire clearly in Fegan's jugular vein—but a clot was also attached to the tip of the wire. With that reading, I told Fegan that the original radiology reading from 2006 had not been an error, and the others weren't, either. Part of the VNS device was indeed in his jugular vein.

At first Fegan refused to believe it. He liked Sullivan, and she had told him the finding was just a mistake. When told the reading had been confirmed and was no mistake, he still rejected the idea, saying, "But I would have bled to death if it was in my jugular vein."

What Fegan didn't realize was that lead wires can penetrate surrounding tissues. Lead-wire problems were well known to

Cyberonics and the FDA, and the agency issued three recall notices for them in 2007, indicating that they were prone to "breakage, corrosion, and dissolution." This could cause them to penetrate surrounding tissues and trigger intense inflammatory reactions with progressive scarring, problems so severe that some surgeons routinely declined to remove the wires, saying it was too dangerous to do so. In one report, a surgeon attempting to remove the wires wrote that not only had a lead wire broken, the patient's vagus nerve had also "disintegrated."

Although the clot in Fegan's jugular vein may never break loose, he knows that if it does, it could pass from his jugular into the right side of his heart and out to his lungs, where it could cause a potentially fatal pulmonary embolus. If the wire were to erode into the carotid artery, which lies adjacent to the jugular vein and vagus nerve, and if a clot broke off inside the carotid artery, it could migrate to the brain, causing a stroke.

But Sullivan remained mum about the findings, never telling Fegan of the danger still lurking in his body from the device he'd had turned off years ago—the device a surgeon said was too dangerous to remove completely. Sullivan told Fegan there was nothing more she could do for him. Her dismissal of him puzzled Fegan, but he decided he'd simply have to find yet another neurologist.

Shortly after Sullivan last saw Fegan, between August of 2013 and December of 2014, she was paid more than two thousand dollars as a speaker for Cyberonics. She was just one of many physician recipients of the company's largesse. Cyberonics spread its love around liberally: records show that during that time period the company paid $2.71 million to 3,456 doctors to promote the VNS device.

No matter where Fegan turned, he was likely to bump into strands of the spiderweb of interlocking economic connections that make up the medical-industrial complex. No wonder that when he went looking for help he couldn't find it.

* * *

Industry largesse, subverting and quietly seducing players across all sectors of the medical-industrial complex, has contributed not only to the rise of corporatized medicine and research but also to a deepening divide among doctors and policy makers about how healthcare and medical research should be organized. Some, like Dr. Eugene Braunwald, embrace academic-industry ties as a way to speed discovery and improve care, while others, like Bernard Lown and Jerome Hoffman, say that leaving healthcare to profiteers raises prices and betrays the trust between patient and doctor.

Braunwald's career exemplifies some of the effects of the transformation of medical research under the pressures of profit seeking. Braunwald had begun his career as a salaried doctor working at the National Institutes of Health, where he made breakthrough discoveries that have withstood the test of time. His extensive contributions in four key areas of cardiology—congestive heart failure, valvular disease, heart attacks, and hypertrophic cardiomyopathy—all came during this period. He wasn't taking out patents or running a research empire with industry funding. He was a salaried academic, driven by what drives all good scientists—intense curiosity and a desire to solve problems. And while he enjoyed public recognition, professional honors, and a good income, he was not on the fast track to grand riches.

But as the decades passed, things began to change for Braunwald, as they did for the entire healthcare system. The new alliance between academia, industry, and venture capitalists had a dual impact on Braunwald's work. On the one hand, it became far more lucrative.[*] On the other hand, for the first time in his career, his work

---

[*] Braunwald says that while he did receive payments from pharmaceutical companies, "Neither I nor my immediate family have owned stocks or stock options in the companies while studying their drugs. Nor did I ever receive salary support from them."

began to be plagued by scandal and questionable science. Unlike Braunwald's earlier research, a number of his contributions during this period would not withstand the test of time.

As we've seen, one of the factors obscuring the truth about medical devices is the increasing scarcity of non-commercial research. In 1977, industry sponsorship of medical research comprised 29 percent of funding. By 2009, that figure had increased to 60 percent, and by 2014, 86 percent of clinical trials were funded by industry.[319] As with other features of the medical-industrial complex, this problem has a complicated history that stretches back several decades.

Back in the 1960s, there was a powerful movement afoot to insulate university-based research from corporate pressures. The unpopularity of the Vietnam War led to massive campus protests against the power of the military-industrial complex. Students and politically engaged citizens, including many academics, demanded that universities distance themselves from doing research for corporate entities. But politicians—themselves often the recipients of funding from the military-industrial complex—fought back fiercely. They not only wanted universities to conduct military research, they also wanted the US to be *the* global leader in scientific and technological innovation. To do that, they believed that universities had to strengthen their ties to industry.

In the 1980s, President Ronald Reagan and his science adviser, George Keyworth, threw their weight behind "technology transfer"—the movement of ideas from academia to the marketplace.[320] A key tool for promoting technology transfer was the Bayh-Dole Act, which promoted university-industry partnerships by allowing universities and their individual researchers to claim patent rights for their innovations. This opened a new funding stream for academia never before possible. The opportunities for profits were dazzling—and medical science was on the front line.

The now defunct Office of Technology Assessment (OTA)

warned against mingling academic research with commercial interests, saying that doing so could "adversely affect the academic environment of universities by inhibiting free exchange of scientific information, undermining interdepartmental cooperation, creating conflict among peers, or delaying or impeding publication of research results."[320] The OTA also cautioned that important research "with no commercial payoff" (such as public health initiatives and basic science) might be abandoned in favor of research that could deliver profits. These warnings were largely ignored in the rush to support university research with potential commercial value.

Congress passed the Bayh-Dole Act on December 12, 1980. Support for the act increased on the heels of a Supreme Court decision, *Diamond v. Chakrabarty* (1980), which ruled that researchers could patent life forms, turning on its head the long-standing assumption that living things could not be covered by patent law. When genetic engineer Ananda Mohan Chakrabarty developed a genetically modified bacterium, the court ruled that he could patent not only the *process* of developing the bacterium but also the actual bacterium itself. In the words of Sheldon Krimsky, professor of urban and environmental policy and planning at Tufts University:[320]

This ruling opened the floodgates for the patenting of cell lines, DNA, genes, animals, and any other living organism that has been sufficiently modified by humans to qualify as "products of manufacture." With this ruling by the Supreme Court, university scientists who sequenced genes had intellectual property that they could license to a company or that could serve as the catalyst for forming their own company.

The Chakrabarty ruling electrified academics and cash-strapped universities. The allure of cashing in on their research was irresistible.

Eugene Braunwald jumped on the Bayh-Dole bandwagon early.

As we've seen, Braunwald was deeply committed to the value of scientific medical research, and he was undoubtedly excited by the availability of funding from industry to support vast new fields of such research. He was also a true believer in the power of academic and business partnerships to promote medical innovation.

In 1978, in what may be one of Braunwald's earliest investigations cosponsored by industry,[*] Braunwald and his coauthors published the results of a study of eight heart failure patients treated with a new drug, amrinone.[321] The study was sponsored jointly by the NIH and Sterling-Winthrop, the manufacturer of amrinone. Braunwald and his colleagues reported that the drug had a "substantial salutary" effect and was well tolerated.

However, British cardiologist Peter Wilmshurst also studied the drug and found that amrinone not only didn't improve heart failure but also "frequently caused life-threatening side effects."[322] When he showed Sterling-Winthrop his results, obtained from a study that used four times the number of patients reported by Braunwald, the company pressured him to exclude certain patients from his analysis. Wilmshurst refused. To do so, he said, would suggest "an apparent but spurious" benefit for patients in heart failure. When Wilmshurst refused to change his analysis, the company threatened him with a lawsuit.[323]

Wilmshurst didn't back down, so Sterling-Winthrop took another tack: it ended Wilmshurst's research on amrinone by removing the drug from the hospital pharmacy and research institute where Wilmshurst conducted his study.[324, 325]

Wilmshurst wondered about Braunwald's glowing review of the drug and looked into the financial interests of Braunwald and his

---

[*] Doctors and medical journals typically did not declare financial conflicts of interest at the time, making it difficult to know exactly when Braunwald first took industry funding for his research or other activities. He has declined to disclose this information.

colleagues. He discovered that not only was the study cosponsored by the manufacturer, as had been reported, but of the five authors who were listed as "employed by the Cardiology Department at Harvard Medical School," two were full-time employees of Sterling-Winthrop and had never worked at Harvard and "[t]wo of the three that worked at Harvard were also paid consultants to the company."[326, 327]

Braunwald was on the editorial board of the *New England Journal of Medicine,* which published his claims, but when Wilmshurst submitted his own findings to the journal for publication, his paper was refused. Although Braunwald may not have played an active role in the publication decision, reputational power may have. Eventually, although some small, uncontrolled studies reported the benefits of amrinone, subsequent controlled studies found that the drug offered no apparent benefit and was associated with significant harms.[328, 329]

Wilmshurst turned over numerous documents to the British newspaper *The Guardian* chronicling the entire affair, including some documents revealing the ruses used by Sterling-Winthrop to suppress negative outcomes related to amrinone.[330, 331] The true profile of amrinone's safety and efficacy remains distorted to this day.

Wilmshurst received the HealthWatch annual award for his work on amrinone, and he was praised for his spine and good humor by Richard Smith, former editor of *The BMJ.*[323]

The amrinone affair was the first apparent crack in Braunwald's credibility. But it was soon followed by other questions about the reliability of his research claims.

In 1981, John Darsee, a researcher in Braunwald's lab, confessed to a single instance of data forgery, but later investigations of his more than one hundred publications revealed that over a period of twelve years he had fabricated much of the data used in those publications. Some eighty-two articles and abstracts were eventually retracted.[332] Thirty of his papers were published while he was at

Harvard working with Braunwald.[333] Four of six articles he coauthored with Braunwald had to be retracted.

Darsee's coworkers had repeatedly voiced their suspicions to their immediate supervisor, Robert Kloner, who notified Braunwald that Darsee was thought to be fabricating data. Braunwald said he conducted an internal investigation and, other than a single episode in which Darsee admitted to faking dates on a report, found no wrongdoing. However, Braunwald didn't report the charges to the NIH, which had funded the research.[334] Darsee's coworkers believed he was so favored by Braunwald that he was essentially untouchable. It was only when coworkers found discarded data in a trash can that they discovered the hard evidence needed to show that Darsee had indeed made up data.[332]

Eventually the NIH was notified and sent investigators to look into the charges against Darsee. They reportedly discovered "a massive fraud": the data for a number of Darsee's published experiments did not exist. This was particularly awkward for Harvard and Braunwald because they had maintained up to that point that during their investigations they had reviewed the data fully.[335]

Two NIH scientists, Walter W. Stewart and Ned Feder, independently got wind of the scandal and decided to examine it further. They wanted to know whether Darsee's forty-seven coauthors—including Braunwald—should have realized that Darsee had fabricated data.[336] When Stewart and Feder eventually published the results of their investigation, they couched their findings in careful language, but the implications were clear: Braunwald had been incautious at best, and at worst he had turned a blind eye to fraud.

Braunwald wasn't about to take the charges lying down. When Stewart and Feder submitted a draft version of their article to Braunwald for his comments, he came out swinging. Bancroft Littlefield Jr., Braunwald's attorney, told Stewart and Feder that their article was "defamatory" and "libelous" and that he would encourage

Braunwald to "take appropriate legal action" if they published the article.

Braunwald's threats worked—for a while. As the targets of Braunwald's wrath, Stewart and Feder were unable to publish their findings for more than three years. Littlefield sent a similarly threatening letter to John Maddox, editor in chief of *Nature,* indicating that the journal, which initially expressed interest in publishing the article, would also be subject to a potential lawsuit. *Nature* backed away.[337]

At least fifteen journals also turned Stewart and Feder's paper down—some explicitly citing the threat of lawsuit.[336] Eventually, however, in 1987, after more than a three-year delay, *Nature* went ahead and published the article.[338] Still, Braunwald's formidable influence was apparent: the article was published with a highly unusual disclaimer. A statement from the *Nature* editors at the end of the article read: "Some editorial changes have been made in this manuscript without the consent of the authors. A reply from Braunwald follows."[338, 339] The publishers appended a lengthy defense by Braunwald in which he said he was "staggered" by the extent of Darsee's fraud but denied Stewart and Feder's charge that Darsee's articles contained "an abundance of errors," inconsistencies, and "lapses from standards" that should have alerted his coauthors.[338] Braunwald dismissed virtually all Stewart and Feder's findings, saying that "allegations involving the papers from Harvard—all of which were retracted in 1982—are insubstantial or simply wrong and have nothing to do with scientific misconduct."[339]

However, in defending his work with Darsee, Braunwald implicitly admitted to a duplicitous presentation of his research with Darsee and Kloner. The trio claimed to have used computer-generated randomization in a study involving the salvage of heart muscle in dogs, but they mixed in historical data to the control group, undermining the authors' claim of scientific rigor. Braunwald acknowledged that they did not reveal the use of historical data in the article but defended their actions, saying they did so to spare the "sacrifice of animals" even though some animals were sacrificed.[340]

Although he denied wrongdoing, certain damage had been done. Braunwald's research claims, once considered golden, were thought by some to be misleading or worse.

Yet many in the world of medicine continued to revere Braunwald, whose research empire was delivering the gold and whose power and influence were spreading around the globe. But the amrinone and Darsee imbroglios were just harbingers of things to come. Although Braunwald conducted industry-sponsored or cosponsored research prior to 1984, in that year he increased his ties to industry by several orders of magnitude when he founded the Thrombolysis in Myocardial Infarction (TIMI) Study Group, which rapidly grew into a multibillion-dollar multinational organization. TIMI studies focused on the use of a clot-buster drug, tPA, which Braunwald studied first as a treatment for blood clots in the lungs, then as a treatment for heart attacks, and subsequently as a treatment for strokes. The drug was the brainchild of Genentech, the world's first biotech company. Braunwald and Genentech would be intimately connected for many years. And despite the early tussles over his research, this was still the 1980s and not a time for skeptics. The entire world was agog with the marvels of modern medicine and the rise of the newest technology: the biotech industry. It was all so hopeful.

* * *

On November 13, 1987, spectators watched fireworks explode on the ground while controllers at the San Francisco International Airport halted overhead air traffic for ten minutes. A perplexed pilot observed, "They don't close airports unless it's for God or Air Force One." But neither God nor Air Force One was arriving at the San

Francisco airport that day. The cause for celebration was, incredibly, a drug. As *Fortune* magazine recounted, the big event was the Food and Drug Administration's approval of tPA.[341] San Francisco, home of Genentech, the biotech company that developed tPA, was set to share in the windfall to come. So it was indeed time for fireworks and celebration. Genentech cofounder and venture capitalist Robert A. Swanson was ecstatic.

Swanson wasn't the only one celebrating. Doctors across the nation had already proclaimed the drug as lifesaving—impressed that a figure no less than Eugene Braunwald, the father of modern cardiology, was hailing tPA as "penicillin of the heart"—a discovery as historic as the advent of antibiotics.[342] Braunwald would play a significant role in promoting tPA as a treatment for heart attacks over an older, cheaper drug, streptokinase.

But tPA's road to FDA approval was not easy. Without Braunwald's backing, it's possible the drug would never have made it to market. Braunwald's cousin Eugene Kleiner was the head of a venture capital firm that invested seed money in Genentech. Braunwald says his cousin played no role in his subsequent involvement with the study of Genentech's clot buster, but introductions weren't necessary; Genentech jumped at the opportunity to have the world's leading cardiologist on its side. It was a relationship that would form the basis for much of Braunwald's research—and the growth of Braunwald's TIMI Study Group. Although initial funding for TIMI came from the National Institutes of Health, it quickly attracted funding from big pharma, device manufacturers, and the biotech industry—particularly from Genentech, which produced TIMI's chief initial drug of study, tPA—though neither Braunwald nor Genentech would reveal the amount of the funding.[343]

Braunwald's partisanship was evident throughout the process of bringing tPA to market. Insider trading rules and clinical-trial ethics rules prohibited Braunwald from telling Genentech (or any outside entity) about the early findings of the TIMI study comparing the clot busters tPA and streptokinase in the treatment of heart attacks. But Genentech was desperate to know; a good deal of money was at stake.

Elliott Grossbard, Genentech's director of clinical research, describes how Braunwald and Genentech got around the prohibition.[342] Braunwald called Grossbard and asked him to come to Boston. Grossbard flew in and met with Braunwald, who peppered Grossbard with questions about how quickly Genentech could produce more tPA. Grossbard interpreted Braunwald's queries as a way of telegraphing the preliminary results to him without doing so directly. Grossbard said, "Braunwald basically leaks to me that the difference [between tPA and streptokinase] is pretty overwhelming in terms of opening up the arteries. I was ecstatic."[342] Grossbard knew that tPA had to be performing well in the TIMI trial or there would be no need to ramp up production.

Braunwald gives a different account of his conversations with Grossbard. He says he simply "needed to understand more about this totally new drug," adding, "If Grossbard thought I was 'telegraphing' anything, he was mistaken..." In fact, says Braunwald, he couldn't have telegraphed the results of the study to Grossbard because he didn't know the results until the trial was stopped early by the board that monitored the study.

Despite Grossbard's excitement after his visit with Braunwald, not everything would go smoothly. At one point, the FDA ordered Genentech to stop testing the drug immediately. The agency discovered that the company was using Chinese hamster ovary cells to produce tPA, and fragments of tumor-causing viruses had been discovered in the cell line.

The timing couldn't have been worse. Other companies were working on competitor products. If Genentech didn't manage to win FDA approval before other companies, it could be left out in the cold. Grossbard flew to Washington, DC, to plead his case with the FDA. He told the agency that an NIH trial—the one conducted by Braunwald—was under way. Grossbard said, "Because it was the NIH and it was this big operation, they backed off," adding, "We had this tremendous gift of being able to dodge bullets."[342]

Genentech was able to keep producing tPA. But the scientific results needed for approval were not forthcoming. The company knew that it was not well positioned going into FDA hearings on May 29, 1987. Streptokinase, an older and far cheaper drug, had been shown to reduce overall deaths by about 20 percent.[344] Genentech and TIMI had only conducted tests of tPA's effect on surrogate markers, such as "time to open vessel," rather than its effect on mortality.

However, Genentech and tPA enthusiasts weren't about to let weak science stand in the way. They somehow managed to persuade *Wall Street Journal* editors to publish, on the day before the FDA advisory meeting, a commentary insisting that tPA should be approved. One of the FDA officers passed out a copy of the editorial at the advisory meeting, saying drily, "Well, it looks like we don't have anything else to do."[342]

Despite their PR effort, FDA advisers voted against approval of tPA. Instead they voted to approve streptokinase.

Then something strange happened.

Despite the vote by the expert medical panel to flunk tPA and approve streptokinase, FDA managers ruled that *neither* drug would be approved. The action, dubbed the Friday afternoon massacre, was a staggering setback for Genentech. Genentech stock values plummeted. Things looked even worse for Genentech when the FDA decided in early November of 1987 to reverse its position and approve streptokinase for the treatment of heart attacks.

But science would be no match for Genentech's PR machine. Patients and cardiologists, influenced by Genentech's PR and/or money, inundated the FDA with demands for the approval of tPA. Talk show host Larry King, who had been treated with tPA for a heart attack, railed against the FDA on his show. Most important, Eugene Braunwald jumped into action and composed a telegram to Senator Ted Kennedy to be signed by other prominent cardiologists. Braunwald's name alone was so powerful that one cardiologist had just one question about the telegram: was Braunwald going to sign it? When told he was, the cardiologist said, "If Gene Braunwald is going to sign that, then I'll sign it, too."[342]

Braunwald's intervention paid off. According to Linda Marsa's book *Prescription for Profits,* Senator Kennedy reportedly spoke with FDA commissioner Frank E. Young, and on November 13, 1987, the FDA announced its approval of tPA for the treatment of heart attacks.

Once the drug was approved, Genentech still had to fight off its chief competitor, streptokinase, in the marketplace. It would be a hard sell: Genentech set the price of tPA at more than ten times the price of streptokinase—about $2,200 for a dose of tPA versus $200 for streptokinase. Genentech had to show that tPA was superior to streptokinase in order to justify the higher price. British cardiologist Peter Wilmshurst says that US cardiologists "made a virtue" of the greater cost of tPA, saying that the high price "was evidence that it was better than streptokinase" and that they told patients, "Greater price must mean better quality."

Initially Braunwald and Genentech claimed that tPA was safer than streptokinase because it was "clot specific" and would break up only the clot causing the heart attack without affecting the normal mechanisms that stop bleeding. And, unlike streptokinase, which was routinely given with the blood thinner heparin, tPA could be given without heparin, which they claimed would make it less likely than streptokinase to cause troublesome side effects, especially bleeding and brain hemorrhage.

But Genentech's safety claim failed to hold up. William R. Bell, the researcher who was testing tPA's clot-specific nature at Genentech's request, didn't find a safety benefit. As he was preparing to submit his findings to the *New England Journal of Medicine*, he came under "big-time pressure" to withdraw the paper. Linda Marsa relates what happened:

> One of his superiors came down to talk to him. "Is there any way that's humanly possible that there might be a mistake?" he asked Bell.
>
> "Well, I'm a human being," Bell responded. "Sure, I can make one. But I don't really think so. These are standard pedestrian-type assays that we're doing—and it's certainly not the first time we've done this."
>
> "Do you think there's even a possibility that these things are wrong?" he pressed.
>
> "Well"—Bell shrugged—"I'm not God."
>
> "Then I think you'd better withdraw this," he was told.
>
> Bell complied.

Other research also failed to support the clot-specific safety claims. In fact, tPA caused *more* strokes resulting from brain hemorrhage than streptokinase did. In a study of nearly 21,000 patients, 1.0 percent of patients treated with streptokinase developed a hemorrhagic stroke following treatment compared to 1.3 percent of patients given tPA.[345] Following challenges to the safety claim, the company changed tack: tPA, it now said, might not be safer, but it was more *effective*. The claim was based on the open-vessel hypothesis, which maintained that tPA opened blocked arteries more quickly than streptokinase did, which they said would mean less heart muscle would be damaged.[346, 347]

Then, in 1985, Braunwald and his colleagues published the results of the landmark TIMI 1 trial in the *New England Journal of Medicine*.[347]

They reported that ninety minutes after treatment, twice as many patients treated with tPA compared to those treated with streptokinase had opening of a blocked coronary artery, which they demonstrated by angiography—shooting dye in the patients' coronary arteries. They concluded that tPA "represents a major therapeutic advance in thrombolysis, having almost twice the thrombolytic effectiveness of intravenous streptokinase with the same or lower incidence of side effects."[347]

Braunwald and his colleagues stopped the study early, after testing just 290 patients, claiming that tPA was so effective that it would have been "unethical" to continue the TIMI trial to completion because it would "deprive" patients of superior treatment.

Jerry Hoffman saw things differently. The New England Journal of Medicine paper, he said, "provided no information about clinical outcomes, so it seemed clear that this was simply another claim based on yet another surrogate marker." What's more, Hoffman pointed out, the paper "didn't answer truly important questions: Does opening the vessels faster actually make a difference in patient outcomes? Will fewer patients die of a heart attack? Or develop congestive heart failure? Or return with chest pain or another heart attack? These are the things that matter to patients—clinically relevant so-called 'patient-oriented' end points—not laboratory measures or physiologic theories that might or might not mean anything."

Hoffman also warned that stopping studies early for presumed benefit is known to increase the risk of bias that contributes to the illusion of benefit where there may be none.[348]

But Hoffman was waving his arms in the dark. The hypothesis that achieving vessel opening at ninety minutes would save lives and preserve heart function was so seductive and logically compelling that most doctors simply didn't question the claim. The chorus supporting Genentech's assertions was growing. The superiority of tPA seemed like a slam dunk. Surely opening a blocked coronary artery earlier had to provide a clinical benefit.

Hoffman says, "When the NIH concludes that the question is so clearly answered that the study doesn't need to be finished, and the *New England Journal of Medicine* agrees that it's important enough to publish the limited results, that attracts a great deal of interest." But, he said, "The claim that tPA was more effective than streptokinase was purely theoretical and not yet verified by patient-oriented outcomes in this or any other study."

Still, few doctors were paying close attention to the science behind tPA. Instead most relied on the recommendations of luminaries such as Braunwald. For them, tPA had proved superior, and its use became almost universal in the US.

Hoffman continued to urge caution. In his lectures, he hammered away at the unproved claims about the putative benefits of tPA. He sent a letter to the NIH pointing out that reliance on surrogate markers and a prematurely stopped study were not sufficient evidence of benefit.

Once again, his cautions were prescient. After the FDA approved tPA, the TIMI researchers gradually published the results of clinically important outcomes (though always in far less prestigious or widely read journals than the *New England Journal of Medicine*), and three years after their 1985 publication announcing tPA's superiority to streptokinase, Braunwald and his colleagues acknowledged that "there was no significant difference" in either mortality or recurrent heart attacks between the two treatment groups.[349]

In light of this, the NIH was forced to reconsider its earlier decision that the superiority of tPA had been proved by the small number of test subjects in the TIMI 1 trial, and they called for a larger head-to-head trial of tPA versus streptokinase to examine clinical outcomes and overall death rates.

This sent Elliott Grossbard into a tizzy. He vehemently opposed such a trial. Genentech, basically a one-trick-pony company that depended almost entirely on tPA for its profits, had already won control of the US market.[350] During a private meeting in Washington, DC, with Braunwald and two of his colleagues, Grossbard argued against a new study: "Almost every cardiologist in America is convinced that tPA is so good that you had to stop the study," he said. "We don't know how another trial would turn out. And if we don't come out ahead, we would have a tremendously self-inflicted wound. So why should we do it?... This could be a good thing for America, but it wasn't going to be a good thing for us."[342]*

Grossbard was right. If tPA did prove superior to streptokinase, it couldn't benefit the company because doctors in the US were already using the drug almost exclusively. But if tPA proved to be no better or even inferior to streptokinase, they could expect to lose, and lose big.

At first Genentech forestalled the head-to-head trial the NIH had demanded by simply refusing to supply tPA. But the company was forced to change its stance after two massive European trials involving approximately sixty thousand patients found no difference between tPA and streptokinase in clinical outcomes.[351, 352] Worse, the studies confirmed that patients treated with tPA suffered more strokes from brain hemorrhage compared to patients treated with streptokinase.[350] European doctors by then were mostly using streptokinase. Facing a growing threat to the US market as a result of the megatrials, Braunwald and a famous University of Michigan cardiologist, Eric Topol, dismissed the European findings, saying they

---

* While attending a journalism conference, I told Linda Marsa, who captured these comments for her book *Prescription for Profits,* that I was amazed that Grossbard would be so blatant about his concern for profits over the public health. Marsa said she had Grossbard's comments on tape—and Grossbard never challenged the published quotations.

were flawed because the researchers didn't give the anticlotting drug heparin with tPA, and the lack of heparin, they said, reduced tPA's efficacy (of course Braunwald and his colleagues had earlier claimed that tPA was safer because heparin wasn't needed with tPA, as it was with streptokinase). Topol wasn't a disinterested expert regarding tPA; at the time, he held options on six thousand shares of Genentech.[353] (Topol eventually had a change of heart, became a critic of drug companies, and called streptokinase the "gold standard drug" for heart attacks.)[354]

In the aftermath of the European trials, advocates of tPA circled their wagons and unleashed scathing attacks on skeptics, leading one cardiologist at the fortieth annual scientific session of the American College of Cardiology to say it was as if any criticism of tPA were "an attack on the American way of life."[354] The vitriol led to some head scratching about why US doctors would cling to a drug that was clearly less safe and more expensive than its rival. Theories ranged from America's love affair with technology to unbridled faith in any new drug made in the US.

Following publication of the European trials in the 1980s, sales of tPA threatened to tank, and Genentech changed its tune. It was now ready to conduct the head-to-head trial the NIH had asked for, but it wasn't about to do it with the NIH. Instead the company would run the trial itself with cosponsors and colleagues around the globe. The study, known as GUSTO (Global Utilization of Streptokinase and Tissue Plasminogen Activator for Occluded Coronary Arteries), was led by Topol, and unlike the European trials it did report a mortality benefit for tPA over streptokinase.

But GUSTO came under strong criticism. Critics pounced on the study, pointing out weaknesses in the study design and "inexplicable" contradictory numbers. Experts in the US and the UK published their doubts, which one critic summed up by saying that the validity of the study was "not clear" but that one thing was "incontrovertible": tPA "is a more dangerous and much more expensive drug than streptokinase."[355, 356]

Jerry Hoffman said, "I believe there are multiple problems with GUSTO, but even if you ignore these, the benefit they claim to have found was tiny. And even that difference goes away if you combine GUSTO's results with those of the two European megatrials."

The crack in Braunwald's reputation appeared to be widening. No longer were doctors automatically buying his claims. According to a *New York Times* report, when Braunwald continued to insist on tPA's superiority to streptokinase at the 1989 annual meeting of the American College of Cardiology, "many cardiologists at the meeting were quick to criticize the study. They said that Braunwald's interpretations far exceeded his data."[357]

★ ★ ★

Braunwald's biographer and fellow Harvard physician, Thomas H. Lee, suggests that Braunwald's insights and research, along with Genentech's development of tPA, were in large part responsible for the dramatic decline in the heart attack death rate, writing, "Since the 1950s, the death rate from heart attacks has plunged from 35 percent to about 5 percent—and fatalistic attitudes toward this disease and many others have faded into history. Much of the improved survival and change in attitudes can be traced to the work of Eugene Braunwald, M.D."[17]

But Jerry Hoffman says that attributing such impressive numbers simply to the effect of treatment relies on yet another illusion. He explains that the death rates cited apparently refer to *case fatality rates*. That is, for every X number of people suffering heart attacks, Y percent die. If one hundred people have heart attacks and twenty of them die, the case fatality, or death rate, is 20 percent. What those numbers don't reveal is how many individuals had a heart attack *overall*—and therefore they don't tell us the *total* number of deaths. In other words, if millions of people suffer heart attacks, and 20 percent of them die, that means a lot of deaths, whereas if thousands of people suffer heart attacks, and 20 percent of them die, that's far fewer deaths. And the number of people diagnosed with a heart attack has increased dramatically in the early part of the twentieth century—not because more people are having serious heart attacks but because increasingly sensitive tests can detect mild heart attacks that would not have been previously diagnosed.

During the first half of the twentieth century, doctors could only identify a heart attack when patients developed symptoms and had changes on their EKGs, or heart tracings. These patients tended to have very severe heart attacks, and case fatality rates were high: up to 35 percent of these patients died.

But in the 1970s, researchers began to refine diagnostic blood tests by identifying enzymes that leak out of damaged heart cells. With each new and increasingly sensitive test, tinier and tinier bits of cellular damage to the heart were identified as "heart attacks." Now, in the twenty-first century, even a patient with a normal EKG tracing and so little heart damage that he or she has no symptoms at all can be diagnosed with a heart attack. These patients tend to be far less likely to die. Adding these patients to the total number of heart attack patients dilutes the pool of symptomatic patients, creating the illusion that fewer people are dying. Before the era of such testing, twenty deaths among one hundred people suffering severe heart attacks (identified by symptoms and EKG changes) meant a 20 percent case fatality rate. Since such testing became widespread, sensitive tests might identify two hundred or even four hundred people as having a heart attack (many with minor or no symptoms), yet still only twenty people die. This slashes the case fatality rate in half, to just 10 percent (or, in the case of four hundred heart attacks, to 5 percent)—even though the overall death rate, or mortality rate, remains the same—creating a fantastic illusion of benefit from clot buster drugs, which happened to come onto the market at the same time that sensitive enzyme tests for heart attacks were developed.

Although increasingly sensitive tests for heart attacks account for a substantial decrease in the case fatality rate, this doesn't explain the whole picture. Total heart attack deaths *have* declined somewhat since approximately 1970, when highly sensitive tests were introduced. However, according to the Centers for Disease Control and Prevention, smoking began to decline in 1968, and that was estimated to account for more than half the decline in deaths, while other lifestyle modifications were responsible for further reductions.

Drugs like tPA can be helpful, but they turn out to account for a very tiny reduction in overall mortality. In fact, tPA offers about the same amount of benefit as a single aspirin: a 2 percent absolute reduction in mortality for the individuals who take the drugs. When aspirin and tPA (or aspirin and streptokinase) are used together, the result is additive, for a 4 percent reduction in death rates. But tPA still carries the pesky side effect of causing brain hemorrhage and can't be used in many heart attack patients, whereas aspirin can be used in most.

But none of this stopped the forward march of Genentech's main money maker or the celebrations that followed the FDA's approval of tPA in 1987, when fireworks exploded and air traffic was stopped. Braunwald and Genentech were celebrating the approval of a drug, yes, but in a larger sense they were celebrating the dawn of a new era, one in which doctors could be multimillionaires and healthcare would come to consume 20 percent of the entire US budget.

In the years to come, those involved in bringing tPA to market would prosper. Herb Boyer, a Genentech cofounder and scientist who helped develop the recombinant-DNA technique used to produce tPA, owned more than two million shares of Genentech stock by 1992—stock valued at $30 million. For his part, Braunwald launched his research empire promoting tPA and ultimately gained substantial funding from Genentech for his research. Meanwhile, it turned out that at least thirteen of the TIMI study authors either owned Genentech stock or held options to buy it at a discount, and none had reported those interests. A congressional subcommittee report determined that "[t]he research literature on t-PA has repeated examples of more positive evaluation of t-PA by scientists with relationships with Genentech, compared to scientists without such relationships." Yet the study carried the blush of independent scholarship, supported by the NIH and led by Eugene Braunwald at Harvard. Genentech stock prices soared from $18 to $28 following publication of the TIMI trial results.

By 2010, the TIMI Study Group trials were almost wholly funded by industry, with some NIH grant support for ancillary studies.[358] Just how much grant money Braunwald's TIMI group would receive from Genentech is secret. When I asked them for the information, Braunwald, the TIMI Study Group, Harvard University, Harvard Medical School, Massachusetts General Hospital, and Genentech all declined to reveal the total amount of funding provided by Genentech for the TIMI trials.

These conflicts of interest led to millions (if not billions) of wasted taxpayer dollars—all in pursuit of a hugely expensive drug that was no more effective and caused more brain hemorrhages than an alternative drug.

Yet Braunwald is unperturbed by the appearance of impropriety. In 2013, I asked him whether he was concerned about conflicts of interest when academic researchers partner with industry. He told me:

This problem has been largely corrected by the development of rigorous disclosure rules, requiring academic investigators to list all of their financial ties to companies with whom they have a working relationship. Most academic institutions now have conflict-of-interest committees which evaluate their faculty's relationships with industry. I think that the problems on the downside are not gone, but I would say it has been reduced by about—I would say by about 90–95 percent.[359]

Braunwald went on to say that academics "have to partner with industry [because] they play a vital role."[339]

While Braunwald claimed that the problem of conflict of interest was 90–95 percent solved, the real-life human toll caused by financial conflicts has continued to mount—at Harvard and elsewhere. And Eugene Braunwald would continue in ensuing years to play a central role in the drama.

* * *

On December 13, 2006, four-year-old Rebecca Riley was found dead after her mother gave her an overdose of prescribed drugs for "bipolar disorder." A public outcry followed Rebecca's death, which raised tough questions about the ethics of diagnosing bipolar disorder in a toddler.[360] There were calls for criminal charges against Rebecca's psychiatrist, Kayoko Kifuji, but Kifuji defended herself, saying she was following the recommendations of Harvard psychiatrist Dr. Joseph Biederman, chief of the clinical and research programs in pediatric psychopharmacology and adult ADHD at Massachusetts General Hospital.

Biederman had almost single-handedly changed pediatric psychiatry by insisting that bipolar disorder could be diagnosed in children as young as two years old, and his work was credited with a fortyfold increase in pediatric bipolar disorder diagnoses. His academic credentials at Harvard gave his recommendations credibility, and doctors and parents alike accepted his recommendations.

An investigation by Senator Charles Grassley found that Biederman failed to disclose that he had received $1.6 million in research funding from fifteen drug companies between 2000 and 2006.[361, 362] Two of the companies, Eli Lilly and Janssen Pharmaceuticals, manufacture two of the antipsychotic drugs he recommended for childhood bipolar disorder, together generating several billion dollars in revenue.[363]

Public outrage over Biederman's role in promoting the drugs led Harvard to form a commission to revise the university's conflict-of-interest policy. Braunwald presided over the commission, and in 2010, after eighteen months of deliberation, he announced changes to the policy that were reported in the media as being "unusually stringent"—even though Harvard researchers could still accept vast sums of industry funding. Although doctors giving talks on behalf of drug companies were prohibited from accepting gifts with a value of $50 or greater, Harvard doctors could still take as much as $5,000 per day for "consulting" with industry under the new "stringent" rules.

There's no doubt that Eugene Braunwald has contributed enormously to scientific and medical knowledge. His stature as one of the leading medical researchers of our time is well deserved. Yet he also embodies some of the most troubling features of the medical-industrial complex. Above all, Braunwald's career illustrates how greatly truth can suffer when the disinterested quest for scientific fact and human benefit becomes interwoven with the drive for profit. And when truth suffers, people suffer.

Chapter Twelve

WHAT IS TO BE DONE?

THE PROBLEMS I'VE DESCRIBED in this book are big and complicated. Fixing them will be a daunting challenge. But it's not impossible. Many brilliant, determined individuals with deep knowledge of the issues are already hard at work on solving them.

One of the leaders of this effort is Bernard Lown. At the age of ninety-five, Lown has a long list of achievements behind him. Along with two colleagues, he identified an abnormal heart rhythm known as the Lown-Ganong-Levine syndrome. As a young cardiologist and researcher at Harvard, he uncovered a critically important link between digitalis, a powerful heart drug, and low potassium, which could cause a deadly reaction.

Lown has also been a lifelong activist. He founded or cofounded nearly half a dozen organizations over the course of his career, including Physicians for Social Responsibility, a national anti–nuclear weapons group, and International Physicians for the Prevention of Nuclear War, for which Lown and his cofounder, then Soviet cardiologist Evgeni Chazov, accepted the Nobel Peace Prize.

But of his many accomplishments, Lown is perhaps best known for leading the effort to develop the modern cardiac defibrillator, which he and José Neuman invented in 1962. Lown had begun working on the device in response to the problem of "sudden cardiac death," a leading cause of mortality in the developed world. Lown realized that, because sudden cardiac death is caused by an electrical failure of the heart and not necessarily by a heart too old or damaged to function, sudden-death patients could be brought back to life.

Before 1962, heart surgeries were rare, and mortality was high. The defibrillator led to the creation of coronary care units where heart attack patients could be watched closely and resuscitated with the defibrillator. The invention also led to a dramatic increase in heart surgeries because doctors had a way to reliably restart hearts they'd paralyzed for surgery.

But over time, Lown would grow increasingly alarmed by the explosive increase in risky and invasive surgeries and other procedures that his invention helped bring about. He strongly suspected that many of these procedures were unnecessary. In the 1970s, Lown proposed a randomized controlled trial to test treatment options for patients suffering from blockages in their coronary arteries. In the test, half the patients would undergo surgery and half would be managed medically. But cardiothoracic surgeons were outraged and declared that such a study would be "unethical." For them, it was obvious that surgery was the only way to treat blocked arteries. Anything less, they assumed, would be malpractice.

Unable to launch the sort of study he wanted, Lown decided instead to study patients who had already been told they needed surgery but who sought a second opinion from him. He published his results in the *New England Journal of Medicine* in 1981.[364] Of 212 men studied for just shy of five years, eleven died (yielding an annual mortality of 1.4 percent), and only nine required bypass surgery. Lown concluded, "There is rarely a need to resort to cardiac surgery;

medical management is highly successful and associated with a low mortality." But his findings were ignored. No one believed them.

Over time, bypass surgeries were replaced by a new treatment: doctors began to implant wire or mesh tubes called stents to prop open the tiny arteries that feed the heart. Each year, 700,000 Americans have coronary-artery stents implanted, according to a report in 2013 by *Bloomberg News*.

As discussed in chapter 4, interventional cardiologists first assumed that these procedures were an improvement over open-heart surgery. But it was an assumption not based on any scientific studies, and Lown wasn't convinced.

He was proved right in 2012, when a meta-analysis of stent implants in 7,229 patients found no benefit in terms of a reduction in future heart attacks or death in patients who had stents placed electively (as opposed to during an evolving heart attack on an emergency basis).[130] Another study confirmed the problem: in 144,737 patients who underwent percutaneous coronary interventions (PCIs), only half (50.4 percent) of the PCIs were found to be "appropriate."[365]

Unfortunately, few heart patients are aware of these sobering statistics. Lown told me about a talk he gave in 2013 to his fellow cardiologists. When he asked them to raise their hands if they told their patients that placing stents in a non-emergency situation would *not* reduce their chances of dying or of having another heart attack. Lown says, "They just hung their heads. No one said a thing."

Lown has come to believe that the most important of all his accomplishments as a physician has been his commitment to educating scores of young cardiologists in the art of "doing as little as possible *to* patients and as much as possible *for* patients." Lown recognized, long before most other physicians, that patients were being subjected to unnecessary treatments and tests—and deprived of the real care they often needed as much as or more than the technological wizardry of modern medicine. He has also come to believe that the problem of overtreatment could help unite people around a new healthcare reform movement by exposing the structural problems underlying a greed-fueled system that betrayed the public health in its drive for profits.

Lown's longtime colleague Vikas Saini, who trained with Lown and became president of the Lown Foundation in 2007, played a role in his decision to focus on overtreatment. After reading journalist Shannon Brownlee's book *Overtreated*, Saini called Brownlee and asked her, "What are we going to do about this?" In a series of conversations, they agreed that many physicians and other healthcare professionals share concerns about the dysfunction of the healthcare system but lack a forum in which to discuss them or develop solutions.

Lown and the nonprofit organization he founded would provide such a forum. In 2012, the Lown Foundation and the New America Foundation, a think tank where Brownlee was working, convened the first meeting ever held on the topic of overtreatment, or unnecessary care. The audience was filled with many luminaries in medicine as well as rank-and-file doctors from around the country and a number of patient activists. Audience members included doctors from Physicians for a National Health Program, the president of the Institute of Medicine, members of the Service Employees International Union, the National Physicians Alliance, women's health groups, and patients' rights organizations. I was there in my role as a medical journalist, sitting alongside Jerry Hoffman, the expert on medical illusions.

As Bernard Lown took his place at the podium, he looked around the airy conference room, taking in each attendee in turn, then said slowly, "Ever since starting clinical practice sixty-two years ago, I have looked forward to this meeting." It was a powerful statement. This lion of medicine was signaling that *this* moment, *this* effort to launch a sustained movement to transform healthcare, was the pinnacle of his life's work. Lown had titled one of his books *Never Whisper in the Presence of Wrong*. On this day, Lown would roar.

His opening statement must have resonated with many of the doctors, nurses, patients, and policy makers in the auditorium that day, who, though each had his or her own reasons for coming, shared a growing disillusionment with medicine, a sense of isolation, and a feeling of frustration with a massive bureaucracy that forces patients through a healthcare system as if they were mere widgets on an assembly line. During conference discussions, clinicians in the room expressed their yearning to connect with their patients and their frustration with the realities of modern healthcare, which force them to check off an increasing number of boxes on a computer, leaving less time to truly listen to their patients. They felt helpless individually to change the situations they face. But this moment, the moment Lown said he'd looked forward to for sixty-two years, was empowering. What one couldn't do, many could.

That moment would mark the birth of a new movement to fix the damage caused by our broken healthcare system. It is a movement that has the potential to radically transform the status quo but that will require profound changes in the culture of medicine and nursing and in society as a whole.

Lown continued, "If more than half a century ago overtreatment was at a trickle pace, it is now at flood tide." He quoted Jerry Hoffman, calling the simultaneous undertreatment of some individuals and overtreatment of others the "Siamese twins of profit-driven medicine." He went on:

High-sounding principles are used by advocates of market-driven medicine to polish its image and are merely incidental.... I believe that the market is not a solution. Indeed it is a major part of the problem. My objection to market-dominated healthcare is on deeper grounds than economic. In a democratic society healthcare must be a right, not a privilege. The underlying issues relate to essential moral principles. At the core...is a covenant of trust between health professionals and patients... [and] the expectation that the patient's needs will be placed first, over and beyond personal interests of the interests of any third party.

There is a moral absolute in medicine to help and never to wrong the patient. No such moral absolute can be found in the marketplace. Caveat emptor, let the buyer beware, is its underlying admonition. The warm and fuzzy rhetoric that "patients come first" is a transparent marketing ploy. For-profit healthcare is essentially an oxymoron.

When Lown finished his speech to thunderous applause, Hoffman turned to me and said in a reverential tone, "He's like Martin Luther King—and many of the people applauding him have no idea just how radical both of them are."

Bernard Lown and his followers aren't the only ones striving to fix the problems created by the medical-industrial establishment. The Mario Negri Institute for Pharmacological Research, founded in 1961 in Italy, was conceived as a way to conduct medical research free of commercial distortions. Its 750 researchers and staff members are all salaried and receive no additional financial rewards for their discoveries. They do not hold patents for their inventions, instead turning over patent rights to manufacturers for one dollar. The institute has been proving for more than half a century that scientists will not only innovate but will also produce some of the most important research in the world without the incentives—or distortions—of profit.

Donald Light, coauthor of *Good Pharma*, a book about the institute, notes that its research into drug treatments for cancer, heart disease, kidney diseases, and many rare ailments as well as its studies of environmental toxins, drug addiction, and epidemiology have won widespread respect. Its carefully constructed heart attack studies, published in the most prestigious medical journals, include one that was responsible for refuting the claim promoted by Braunwald and other industry advocates that the expensive new clot buster tPA was superior to streptokinase for the treatment of heart attacks.[351, 366]

Free of commercial pressures, Mario Negri researchers can do what industry-sponsored researchers generally can't or won't do. In Light's words, "They can research any active ingredient that might help with a disease whether it is patentable or not." They can also conduct head-to-head trials of drugs to determine which is superior for a particular condition, including studies that compare older, cheaper drugs to newer, more costly offerings.

Since institute researchers are insulated from market forces, they are also free to research environmental toxins without fear of retaliation from corporate sponsors. In the wake of a huge chemical explosion in Italy in 1976, cabbages, turnips, and cats were found to be dying of an unknown cause. Negri researchers were able to trace the problem to dioxin, a chemical then being produced by the pharmaceuticals company Roche that is related to Agent Orange. However, the institute does accept up to (but no more than) 10 percent of its budget from industry—with non-negotiable conditions usually not required by contract research organizations. According to the institute's director, Silvio Garattini, these conditions require that the institute must be solely responsible for the planning and conduct of any study and that "ownership of the data and any decision made regarding their publication belongs to the researchers without any influence from the company." These strict rules led one company to back out, unwilling to grant full independence to the institute.[367]

During the first two decades of the twenty-first century, other groups of professionals and activists dedicated to reforming the healthcare system have emerged. By 2016, the "new civil rights movement for healthcare" that Lown envisioned was beginning to take shape. Many leaders of this new movement gathered that year in Chicago at the fourth annual conference of the Right Care Alliance, a project founded by the Lown Institute that welcomes all groups and individuals committed to healthcare reform, from labor unions to doctors' groups to patient safety organizations.

Some speakers focused on the ways medical overtreatment in the US tends to crowd out other forms of social spending. For example, Lauren Taylor, a PhD student at Harvard Business School and coauthor of *The American Health Care Paradox,* explained that for every dollar spent on healthcare, the US spends only ninety cents on social welfare programs such as those that offer job training, housing, and nutritional counseling. By contrast, other wealthy nations belonging to the Organisation for Economic Co-operation and Development (OECD) spend two dollars on social welfare for every dollar spent on medical care—and enjoy longer life expectancies and lower infant mortality rates than the US does.[368]

Other speakers analyzed the social disparities in US healthcare and described programs that could help reduce them. Jeff Brenner, a family physician and executive director of the Camden Coalition of Healthcare Providers, in Camden, New Jersey, recounted his experiences working in a poor Puerto Rican and Dominican community beset by violence: "Primary care is utterly failing. We run from room to room to room in meaningless increments of meaningless fifteen-minute visits." Brenner found that his patients, "swept in and out of a vortex of chaos," were experiencing chronic stress that could lop twenty years off their lives. Under these circumstances, "right care" means changing living conditions. So Brenner and his group raised money to put people with highly complex medical problems into new apartments with a variety of social supports. Not only did their health improve, but costs also went down. (Brenner was profiled by writer and surgeon Atul Gawande in the 2011 *New Yorker* article "The Hot Spotters.")[369]

A number of speakers at the Right Care conference emphasized the need for a broad-based popular movement comparable to the civil rights movement of the 1960s to combat the complex economic and social problems affecting US healthcare. Urban planner and political scientist Phil Thompson recalled growing up "in a family and a network of churches very involved in the civil rights movement" and said that, for the healthcare reform movement to succeed, change must first take place among the people trying to make the change. "The real knowledge leaders are the people who live in the community…but we can't build a movement if everyone shrinks when a doctor walks in a room."

Eliseo Medina, an immigrant from Mexico who went to work after eighth grade picking grapes and worked with Cesar Chavez for eighteen years in the California farm workers movement, called healthcare an essential element of social justice that demands the same sort of mass action farm workers had to take. He said although Obamacare "is an achievement over what we had…it falls far short of what is needed. Far too many people still don't have care." He urged the audience to "discuss strategies and to plan for change," adding that "the road will be long and hard, and it will seem you'll never reach your destination. But if you persevere, there will be victories along the way."

Shannon Brownlee and Vikas Saini, as cochairs of the Right Care Alliance, know that one of their jobs is to lay out a strategy for a better system—and a vision for what that system would be like both for patients and the people who work within it. They have a "grand strategy," a term they've borrowed from foreign policy experts for a system that integrates healthcare with public health and a concerted national effort to improve health not only with proper medical care, but through social, agricultural, and jobs policies, a strategy, they hope, will serve as a road map for the Right Care Alliance's campaigns.

It isn't clear whether the Right Care Alliance will succeed—or even last. But it represents the kind of union among professional leaders, economic and technical experts, and social and political activists that will be necessary to effect systemic changes to the current system of market-driven medicine.

* * *

One change that would go a long way toward simultaneously reducing undertreatment and overtreatment as well as reducing costs is the establishment of a single-payer health insurance program, sometimes dubbed Medicare for all, in the US. This is the kind of health coverage already routinely provided to citizens of most developed countries. In countries with national health plans, polls show that citizens are happier with their healthcare than their counterparts in the US are—and that their health outcomes and life spans surpass those of US citizens, with a far lower price tag.[370, 371]

In the US, patients complain that they are rushed through their doctor visits as if they were on an assembly line, a problem that arises in large part because the US system requires doctors to track and code every single diagnosis, lab test, and action for billing purposes. Time-motion studies show that US doctors spend more than two hours in administrative tasks for every one hour actually seeing patients and as many as one of every five hours doing purely billing-related tasks.[372, 373] Doctors in England, Canada, and other well-off nations, freed of the burden of tracking every action for billing purposes, can spend less time doing administrative work and more time with their patients.

The French healthcare system provides every citizen with a card that looks much like a credit card and has his or her entire medical record embedded in it, including information from every healthcare provider who sees the patient. Because the patient carries the card with him or her, there are no delays or duplicate test orders because one doctor doesn't have the record from another doctor. Tanya Blumstein, an American, describes the difference between the care she received in the US and the care she received in France as an expectant mother. She says care in the US was "hellish" because she had trouble getting insurance (pregnancy was considered a preexisting condition), and when she did get insurance, she had to work her way through expensive premiums, a high deductible, copays, coinsurance, and out-of-network costs. When she was pregnant in France, she could simply show up at a neighborhood health clinic at any time, with or without an appointment. When her baby was born and became sick with the flu, a doctor came to her home at 3:00 a.m. on a Sunday—all paid for by French public healthcare. During the first week after she gave birth, a nurse came to help with any needs she might have, a service provided to all new mothers in France.[374]

France has one of the lowest infant mortality rates in the world.

Consider, by contrast, the role that our current dysfunctional system of private health insurance has played in limiting access to care, through its extraordinary complexity and expense, and accommodating overtreatment. The latter point may seem counterintuitive, but by leaving everything to the marketplace rather than making rational allocations based on the needs of each community, the insurance industry has promoted the rise of the for-profit medical device industry that led to Dennis Fegan's ordeal. Insurers paid for the VNS device, just as they paid for the treatment of thousands of patients who were hurt by the off-label use of spine implants, unnecessary stents, ASR XL hip implants, and many other flawed devices and procedures.

Contrary to public perception, commercial insurance not only fails to control medical costs in general, it often helps drive overtreatment. Competition among commercial insurers and cost-plus reimbursement schemes, in which insurers receive a percentage of any contracts to cover patient care means that insurers benefit from offering coverage of big-ticket items such as costly medical devices. Insurers pay for these items partly to compete with the offerings of other insurers and partly because the bigger the overall healthcare pie, the bigger their slice of it. In other words, a slice of a several thousand dollar contract covering employees for only minor care would reap little profit compared with a slice of a multi-billion dollar contract covering heart surgery (necessary or not) and organ transplants.

Commercial insurers create massive administrative waste, and they contribute to the preferential treatment of well-insured patients over others. David U. Himmelstein, professor of public health at the City University of New York and a visiting professor at Harvard Medical School, says that insurers have every incentive to "promise the world while delivering as little as possible." So while insurers will cover big-ticket items such as coronary stents (because that's where the money is), they will use every tool available to block or deny coverage on an individual basis after they've won a contract to provide insurance to an individual or a group of employees. Denial of coverage is achieved with a variety of small-print exclusions in policies that leave patients holding the bag.[375, 376, 377]

The American system of paying physicians for specific services provides an incentive for the use of medical devices, whether they are effective or not. Patients have been charged as much as $100,000 for VNS implants, including the price of the device itself, the surgeon's fees, and hospital charges. And doctors have a regular, reliable income as patients return for scheduled checks of and adjustments to their VNS devices, each visit costing several hundred dollars. The allure of substantial financial gain inevitably tempts doctors to take the device company's claims at face value rather than questioning them. Doctors paid with a salary would have no financial motive to perform needless surgeries or implant devices of questionable value. Conversely, a single-payer system eliminates the perverse financial incentives for insurers to reward doctors and their institutions for "saving" money by doing less for certain patients.

Medicare for all, or a single-payer system in which doctors are salaried, could ease or eliminate each of these problems. It would reduce overtreatment by removing financial rewards to doctors for doing more while tackling the problem of undertreatment by providing everyone with access to care.[*] And because everyone would be covered under the same plan, a single-payer system would eliminate preferential treatment of patients based on tiered insurance plans. And a single-payer plan would still allow the availability of additional private insurance for individuals who choose to pay for add-on or "boutique" benefits.

Pundits and politicians often claim that Americans simply won't accept single-payer universal healthcare. Yet polls from the Kaiser Family Foundation, Gallup, and others consistently show that a majority of the US population supports the idea of Medicare for all.[378, 379] And, depending on the poll, roughly half or more of doctors also favor some form of a single-payer system, either along with the option for private insurance or without it.

The patent system, which provides enormous bonanzas for companies that develop and successfully market high-priced medical devices, is also ripe for reform. Patent protection for valuable inventions was developed to encourage and reward scientific creativity.

---

[*] Putting doctors on salary eliminates financial incentives to order more tests (or implant more devices). At the same time, a single-payer system removes pressure from insurers to do less or deny services. Instead the only consideration would be what each doctor believes is best for his or her patient—not how the treatment affects the doctor's income.

But in recent years, the system has been so exploited that it is now obstructing rather than assisting innovation. Patents discourage open sharing of ideas, and because patents are awarded for trivial changes to preexisting items, monopoly extensions have become commonplace—with no benefit to the public. Dean Baker, an economist and codirector of the Center for Economic and Policy Research, in Washington, DC, estimates that getting rid of drug-company patent monopolies would save $270 billion annually in drug costs.

The goals of the system are further subverted by patent trolls—individuals or companies that amass patent rights with no intention of producing—or even the ability to produce—the product patented. Instead they file for patents with the sole intent of suing companies for infringement when they attempt to actually produce the items. This proves profitable for the patent trolls, because companies will often agree to a settlement rather than take on long and costly court battles. A study at Boston University found that patent trolls have drained the US of $500 billion since 1990.

Furthermore, industry often uses research developed on the public dime for private gain. Patents that are developed at taxpayer expense should belong to the public. Free-market advocates often oppose changes to the patent system on the grounds that new discoveries will grind to a halt unless profit incentives are maximized. But the experience of the Mario Negri Institute suggests otherwise. So does history. Scientists have always been driven to their discoveries by intense curiosity—not the promise of profits. Galileo, Einstein, Edward Jenner, Alexander Fleming, John Snow, Ignaz Semmelweis, and many others made seminal contributions to medicine and science without patents or the promise of profits. Sometimes they revealed their discoveries at great expense to themselves, including banishment and loss of livelihood (Semmelweis) and even the threat of death (Galileo).

Some great innovators even actively rejected the patent concept. George Washington Carver, the brilliant agricultural scientist, dismissed the idea that he should patent his hundreds of medical and scientific contributions, saying, "God gave them to me. How can I sell them to someone else?" Similarly, when Jonas Salk was asked in 1955 by newsman Edward R. Murrow who owned the patent on the polio vaccine, Salk replied, "Well, the people, I would say. There is no patent. Could you patent the sun?"

The assumption that only financial incentives can promote innovation ignores giants like Eugene Braunwald, who made his most significant contributions in his early years, while on salary, and Bernard Lown, who developed some of the most important scientific advances of the century while on salary. And it ignores the vast wasteland of patents that boost prices and protect extended monopoly rights on products based solely on minor tweaks that produce little or no public benefit.

Not only will scientists pursue innovative ideas without added financial incentives, but psychological and management studies also repeatedly show that financial incentives can actually inhibit creativity and innovation. In a series of studies sponsored by the Federal Reserve, economists at MIT, the University of Chicago, and Carnegie Mellon University found that financial incentives interfered with test subjects' performance in solving cognitive problems.[380] Their conclusion? Pay people enough money to take the issue of money off the table and allow them to focus on the creative task at hand.[380]

A third element of the healthcare system that is in desperate need of reform is the FDA. Yes, the agency continues to play a vital role in protecting the American public, ensuring that our food and many of our drugs are far safer than the food and drugs in some other countries. But as we've seen, in too many cases the FDA has abdicated its role as watchdog over industry to serve instead as an ally and partner with industry. The FDA claims that its partnerships with industry, through projects such as the joint writing and promotion of the 21st Century Cures Act, promotes innovation. But the FDA cannot be a partner and a watchdog at the same time. The roles must be distinct. To that end, leadership at the FDA must be returned to civil servants—and the practice of putting political appointees in leadership roles should end. In order for the hardworking and brilliant public servants at the FDA—people like the FDA Nine; David Graham, who first sounded the alarm about Vioxx; Andrew Mosholder, who reported on the dangers of antidepressant drugs for adolescents; and others—to do the job they believe in and want to do, agency leadership must be returned to civil servants, and Congress must prohibit political appointments to the agency.

Congress also needs to double the budget of the FDA, as recommended by the Project on Government Oversight, and roll back industry funding of the agency through channels such as the Prescription Drug User Fee Act and the Reagan-Udall Foundation.[381]

The 21st Century Cures Act needs to be drastically changed or abandoned. Lowering the levels of evidence necessary for industry to win FDA approval of its products will mean even worse outcomes for the public than those we are already seeing. The public may assume that deregulation means unburdening industry so it can be more "efficient," but what does efficiency mean? The current administration promises to slash drug and device prices, but it appears that this will not be accomplished by putting caps on industry's exorbitant profits. Instead manufacturers are relying on the president's promise to slash regulations governing device and pharma companies "by 75 to 80 percent," reducing prices by speeding approval times.[382] But that approach doesn't guarantee that any savings will be passed along to the public. Worse, by eliminating regulations intended to ensure scientific testing of devices, we can expect to see an increasing number of untested, unregulated devices pouring onto the market and into our bodies.

To prevent future disasters involving high-risk implanted devices, the FDA should insist that such devices be subjected to at least two randomized, controlled clinical trials that include medically managed control groups as well as sham-device groups whenever possible to control for the placebo effect.[123] Patient-oriented clinical outcomes rather than surrogate end points must be tested, and the agency should seek out non-industry experts and methodologists as advisers.[155, 383, 384]

Needed reforms include the enactment of legislation to restore the right of patients to sue if they are harmed by devices, and Congress should be urged to pass the Sunshine in Litigation Act, which would ensure that important information uncovered during product liability suits isn't held secret under confidentiality agreements. In many instances, drug companies settle cases with injured patients under a provision forbidding the patients' attorneys from notifying the FDA that the drug or device caused harm.[385–388]

These urgently needed reforms have been and continue to be forcefully opposed by industry. Of course, this raises the even bigger problem of industry influence over members of Congress and other politicians, including the president. In the long run, it will not be possible to achieve the changes needed to fix our healthcare system without instituting campaign finance reform and thus eliminating the hold industry has over politicians.

As I've mentioned, another major problem with US healthcare is the lack of sound, independent scientific research. Too often what masquerades as science is not. And mere transparency is not enough: disclosure of the financial ties that connect researchers and regulators to big corporations cannot itself ensure unbiased research. We need to stop the flow of money from industry to public agencies like the FDA, the Centers for Disease Control and Prevention, and the National Institutes of Health (NIH) and replace it with public funding.

Academia, which should be the real engine of independent research, has also been corrupted by lucrative partnerships with industry. We need to recall the reasons why universities came into existence in the first place. In his book *Science in the Private Interest,* Sheldon Krimsky writes that the concept of academic freedom, or "protected employment" of professors from external interests, "has its roots in the Middle Ages, when medieval scholars 'sought to be autonomous and self-regulating to protect knowledge and truth from corrupt outside influences.'" Krimsky goes on to observe that "public-interest science requires people who are able and willing to speak out candidly and critically about toxic dangers, political injustice, pernicious ideolog[ies] that foment hatred, false idols, unsustainable paths of economic development, product liability, and environmental causes of disease."[320]

To protect the lofty goal of encouraging rigorous inquiry without fear or favor, we must insist that our colleges and universities once again function as centers that seek truth, not profit. That means we need to demand that Congress repeal the Bayh-Dole Act and truly insulate our academic centers from industry pressures.

Furthermore, public health policy in the US needs to be modified to deemphasize paying for medical interventions designed to fix health problems and instead stress investment in social programs that can help prevent such problems in the first place. As part of this effort, we need to address the wealth gap, which is the single most powerful predictor of life span. While the most potent cancer drugs, costing between tens of thousands and hundreds of thousands of dollars per person per year in many instances, often add only months to a patient's life span, being on the wrong side of the wealth gap lops up to twenty years off an individual's life in the US.[389–393]

Between 1900 and 2000, life expectancy in the US jumped from forty-seven to seventy-seven years. Many people assume that the thirty-year increase was the result of breakthroughs in modern medicine. But when physician Thomas McKeown studied US mortality rates from the 1700s through the 1900s, he found that 92 percent of the decline in mortality occurred before 1950—the date when the most significant medical advances began to appear. Major increases in life span were the result of declining death rates from eleven infectious diseases, including tuberculosis, pneumonia, and smallpox. And the declines in these diseases actually had less to do with the advent of medicines such as streptomycin and isoniazid than with public health measures, improved housing, and better living standards.[391] Beginning in the 1900s, water chlorination and other drinking-water treatments—along with improved sewage disposal, enhanced food safety, organized solid waste disposal, and public education about hygienic practices such as food handling and hand washing—had a strong impact on reducing deaths.[391]

What's more, medical care does little to explain the dramatic fifteen-to-twenty-year life-span gap between rich and poor that has continued and widened in the US beginning in the latter part of the twentieth century.[390, 394] Sir Michael Marmot, professor of epidemiology at University College London, studied male British civil servants living in Whitehall in the 1970s. After analyzing data about their risk factors for coronary artery disease, he discovered that the higher the man's social position, the longer he lived. The correlation was in direct proportion to each man's position in the bureaucratic hierarchy: the number one official was less likely to have a heart attack than the number two official, the number two official was less likely than the number three official, and so on down the line. Men at the lowest employment grade were four times more likely to have a heart attack than those at the highest grade—and these differences were independent of factors like smoking, serum cholesterol levels, and blood pressure.[389]

A short ride on the Washington, DC, Metro was all it took for Marmot to illustrate the degree of these effects in America.

Traveling from downtown's Union Station to the suburb of Bethesda, Maryland, Marmot demonstrated that each mile traveled was associated with a gain of 1.5 years of life expectancy, which ultimately accounted for a twenty-year difference in life span between the inner city and the affluent suburbs.[394]

This disparity doesn't just harm those at the bottom—it harms everyone. British society is less economically unequal than that of the US, as measured by the income gap between pay for CEOs and pay for the lowest-paid worker. When Marmot compared the two societies, he found that the "better-off Americans had more illness than the better-off English . . . and nearly as much illness as the worst-off English."

The problem of income inequality is highly complex, and proposing a solution to it is beyond the scope of this book. But there are many social programs that have proved to mitigate the factors that lead to poor health outcomes for disadvantaged people. They include early childhood education programs such as Head Start, reliable child-care programs for working families, nutrition programs, prenatal and postnatal care for mothers, and many others. Most are inadequately funded, and many are under constant pressure in the name of "fiscal responsibility" and "personal self-reliance." Making a real national commitment to supporting such programs and making them available to all who need them would have a measurable impact on the health of Americans—and save billions in medical costs.

Such a change in attitude is not a matter of altruism. The welfare and health of our neighbors is central to our own well-being and that of our nation, whether in terms of our ability to protect ourselves from the spread of infectious diseases or industry's need for a healthy workforce.

As a nation, we have agreed to designate certain things that benefit the whole society as common goods. They include basic education, roads and other infrastructure, clean air and drinking water, and services like firefighting and policing. These common goods produce a level of civilization that makes life in America worth living for all citizens. Healthcare should be added to this list. And just as we expect police officers and firefighters to risk their lives for fair salaries, we should expect physicians and medical researchers to work for a fair salary and thus be insulated from the biasing effects of lucre—and to truly work for the common good.

As a young medical-school graduate in the early 1970s, Jerry Hoffman made a decision that was highly unusual at the time: he declined a lucrative offer to give talks around the country for a drug company. In the 1970s, doctors who spoke on behalf of drug companies weren't just highly respected, they were also often revered as the brightest boys on the block. Many were honored speakers at grand rounds and at international conferences and were very well paid with red-carpet perks.

Hoffman turned all this down. He explains, "I've always thought that for a physician, being professional means you have to put your patients' needs first, before your own. As I thought about this offer to join a speakers bureau, I realized that doing so would cripple my ability to make impartial judgments about drugs or research. It became crystal clear to me that I couldn't ever take money or gifts from a drug company without violating the core obligation of my profession."

In Hoffman's view, doctors can't take money and stay unbiased—and a doctor who takes money from industry is no different from a judge who takes money from an attorney who wants to influence the outcome of a case. "It would be considered a bribe in the courtroom," Hoffman says, "yet it's entirely accepted in medicine."

The underlying problem is the fact that we insist upon treating healthcare as a commodity rather than a common good. This philosophy encourages hospitals, medical groups, insurance companies, pharmaceuticals makers, device manufacturers, and other healthcare businesses to put the pursuit of profits ahead of the public welfare. It also encourages ostensibly independent entities, from individual healthcare providers to universities, research institutes, professional associations, scientific journals, and regulatory agencies, to take money from industry, which inevitably biases their judgment.

Most fundamentally of all, we need to agree on a new national attitude toward healthcare—one that considers healthcare as a fundamental human right rather than a privilege reserved for those who can afford to buy it.

Hubert Humphrey, in his last speech as vice president, said, "The moral test of government is how that government treats those who are in the dawn of life, the children; those who are in the twilight of life, the elderly; those who are in the shadows of life, the sick, the needy, and the handicapped."

That same test applies not just to government but also to all of us. For as long as we continue to accept the commoditization of medicine in the name of free markets, then Lown's and Hoffman's vision of a healthcare system that is dedicated solely to the good of patients will remain out of reach.

★ ★ ★

Dennis Fegan's younger son, Derrick, remembers years ago, when he was a teenager, watching when the entire Corpus Christi fire department came out to honor his dad at his retirement ceremony. Derrick was impressed by the camaraderie and respect shown to his father. He knew his dad would miss his buddies and his work as a paramedic and firefighter.

Two decades later, after all the tribulations brought on by his struggle with the effects of the VNS device implanted in him and his battles for recognition, honesty, and restitution by the American medical system, Derrick's dad is back to the quiet rhythm of uneventful days at home. He still has brunch on Sunday mornings at the Town & Country Café. He putters in his yard. He enjoys it when his sons, Derrick and Michael, come to visit from time to time.

But too much has changed. Fegan's family has seen him transformed from an outgoing, active man to a virtual recluse. Now an accountant living in Austin, Michael recalls the changes that occurred over time in his dad. He says that when his father was first released from the hospital after being treated for asystole, he was just happy to be alive. But after learning about the cause of his asystole and encountering an indifferent and dishonest medical establishment, he grew angry. His father began peppering everyone in his network, including family members, with e-mails about the dangers of the VNS device.

Now that his anger has been transformed into ongoing efforts to seek change, Fegan tries not to worry about the VNS wire in his jugular vein or think about the clot that could detach and cause a pulmonary embolus and kill him at any moment. Or, worse, leave him crippled and dependent on others for his daily needs.

Reaching out to the world in the one way he can, Fegan continues his lonely work. He doesn't earn any money for it. He can't win anything for himself. But he can, maybe, help others.

The same desire that led him to become a firefighter and paramedic continues to motivate him, keeping him at his computer surveying the FDA data on the VNS device long after all hope for his own case has been destroyed. Fegan will receive no restitution, not even an apology. He continues to scan the medical literature and scrutinize the MAUDE database, updating other people with epilepsy by posting his findings on the VNS message board. He keeps looking for the right piece of information, the right person or agency that will help protect others from the device that nearly killed him—a task that has become even more important to him since he learned that the military is experimenting with the VNS device as a potential way to treat traumatic brain injuries and post-traumatic stress disorder, among other problems, in soldiers returning home from war.[395, 396]

Mike recalls when his dad's passion for the cause was at its height. "For a while, I got eight to ten e-mails a day. They would be little short e-mails, or just links. After a while, I was like, 'I get it.' But then one day I actually read some of the material, and I thought, wow, he's on to something. I think if it saves even just one life, it's worth it."

Dennis Fegan's sons understand that, although he can no longer go out on ambulance calls as a paramedic and firefighter, their father is still fighting to save lives.

And he's still the hero they looked up to as kids.

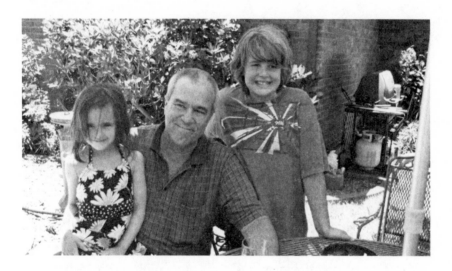

Dennis Fegan with his grandchildren. (Photograph courtesy of the Fegan family)

Industry-Independent Organizations, Publications, and Patient Advocacy and Support Groups

RESOURCES FOR PATIENTS AND HEALTHCARE PROVIDERS

- *Advocating Safety in Healthcare E-Sisters*: U.S.-based online group with a special focus on Essure implants
  http://www.ashesnonprofit.com/
- *Alliance for Human Research Protection*: "Advancing Honest and Ethical Medical Research" (USA)
  www.ahrp.org
- *Breast Cancer Action*: An "independent voice [and] activist watchdog organization" (USA)
  http://bcaction.org
- *Breast Cancer Action Quebec*: "The only independent breast cancer organization in Canada whose mission is to work for the prevention of breast cancer and the elimination of environmental toxicants linked to the disease" (Canada)
  http://www.bcam.qc.ca/
- *Campaign Zero*: Offers "quick information and checklists" to help patients and their families avoid being harmed in the hospital (USA)
  http://www.campaignzero.org/

- *Canadians for Vanessa's Law*: Promotes the Protecting Canadians from Unsafe Drugs Act (Canada)
  Contact David Carmichael at carmichaeldf@gmail.com
- *The Carlat Psychiatry Report*: "An eight-page monthly newsletter (in both print and online form) that provides clinically relevant, unbiased information on psychiatric practice. We receive no corporate funding, which allows a clear-eyed evaluation of all available treatments" (USA)
  www.thecarlatreport.com
- *Center for Medical Education*: "Committed to providing the highest standard in continuing medical education since 1977." Includes lectures and commentary by Jerome Hoffman, among others, in primary care and emergency medicine (USA)
  https://courses.ccme.org/
- *Citizens for Patient Safety*: "Improving health literacy and engaging and empowering patients and families to manage their own health" (USA)
  http://www.citizensforpatientsafety.org/
- *Cochrane Collaboration*: Provides meta-analyses and systematic reviews. Cochrane fails to be as fully industry-independent as its guidelines suggest, and some of its recommendations appear compromised as a result, but many provide the highest-quality evidence and analyses available in multiple languages (UK)
  http://www.cochrane.org/
- *Device Events*: Uses the FDA's adverse-events database reaching back twenty years (USA)
  www.deviceevents.com
- *Essure Procedure*: Online support and advocacy for women harmed by Essure, hosted by Erin Brockovich (USA)
  http://essureprocedure.net/
- *Foundation for Integrity and Responsibility in Medicine*: Publishes *Health Care Renewal*, a blog that provides superb clinical and

policy analyses focused on distortions created by conflicts of interest (USA)

http://www.firmfound.org/

http://hcrenewal.blogspot.com

- gtprevencaoquaternaria's Blog: Brazil. "We are an industry-independent group, mainly working on quaternary prevention."
gtprevencaoquaternaria@googlegroups.com
http://blogdoduro.blogspot.com

- *Harding Center for Risk Literacy*: Germany. Excellent group that "researches, develops and disseminates tools" that clearly explain the risks vs. harms of medical interventions.
hardingcenter@mpib-berline.mpg.de
www.harding-center.mpg.de

- *Health Action International*: "Global network of independent experts in 70 countries share information and expertise in all areas of pharmaceutical policy, including intellectual property, pharmaceutical R&D, free trade, pharmaceutical marketing, clinical trial data transparency and pharmaceutical pricing [so] all people [can] receive the right medicine … at a price they can afford."
http://haiweb.org

- *HealthWatch*: Quarterly newsletter originally focused on unproved treatments that "now promotes evidence and integrity in all forms of medicine and healthcare" (UK)
https://www.healthwatch-uk.org/about/about-healthwatch.html

- *Healthy Skepticism*: Focuses on "reducing harm from misleading drug promotion." Has a superb collection of journal articles and information on a variety of topics, including conflicts of interest, and has a global membership (Australia)
http://www.healthyskepticism.org/global

- *KCE Belgian Health Care Knowledge Centre*: Available in multiple languages (Belgium)
http://kce.fgov.be/

- *Live Life Mesh Free*: Online discussion group for individuals living with surgical mesh implants (USA)
https://www.facebook.com/groups/545418218970988/
- *Lown Institute*: "We seek to catalyze a grassroots movement for transforming healthcare systems and improving the health of communities" (USA)
https://lowninstitute.org/
- *Manufacturer and User Facility Device Experience (MAUDE)*: The FDA's medical device adverse events database (USA)
https://www.accessdata.fda.gov/scripts/cdrh/cfdocs/cfmaude/search.cfm
- *Mothers Against Medical Error*: "Supporting victims of medical harm" (USA)
http://www.mamemomsonline.org/
- *National Physicians Alliance*: "Advancing the Core Values of the Medical Profession: Service, Integrity, and Advocacy" (USA)
http://npalliance.org/
- *National Women's Health Network*: "Improves the health of all women by developing and promoting a critical analysis of health issues in order to affect policy and support consumer decision-making" (USA)
https://nwhn.org/
- *No Gracias*: "Independent civil organization for transparency, integrity and equity in health policy, healthcare and biomedical research." "Organización civil independiente por la transparencia, la integridad y la equidad en las políticas de salud, la asistencia sanitaria y la investigación biomédica." (Spain and Spanish-speaking countries)
http://nogracias.eu/
- *Nordic Cochrane Centre*: See *Cochrane Collaboration*, above (Denmark)
http://nordic.cochrane.org/

- *Physicians for a National Health Program*: "Non-profit research and education organization of 20,000 physicians, medical students and health professionals who support single-payer national health insurance" (USA)
  http://www.pnhp.org/
- *Prescrire*: "Independent information on treatments and health-care strategies," available in French and English (France)
  http://english.prescrire.org/en/Summary.aspx
- *ProPublica Patient Safety Community*: Online forum for "constructive dialogue about patient harm, its causes and possible solutions" (USA)
  https://www.facebook.com/groups/patientharm/?fref=nf
- *Right Care Alliance*: "A coalition to stand up for what healthcare should be," addressing both undertreatment and overtreatment and advocating for "right care" (USA)
  http://rightcarealliance.org/
- *RxISK*: "Free, independent drug safety website to help you weigh the benefits of any medication against its potential dangers" (UK)
  https://rxisk.org/
- *Safe Patient Project*: Advocacy arm of Consumers Union (USA)
  http://safepatientproject.org/
- *The NNT*: Free evidence reviews using only "the highest quality, evidence-based studies (frequently, but not always Cochrane Reviews), and we accept no outside funding or advertisements" (USA)
  http://www.thennt.com/
- *Therapeutics Initiative*: "Independent Healthcare Evidence"; provides excellent evidence reviews (Canada)
  http://www.ti.ubc.ca/
- *Unplugged Health and Medicine*: Part of the "Quarternary Prevention Movement's purpose is to work together to create health

and well-being." (Cuba, Peru, Colombia, Chile, Uruguay; posts also available in English)

https://seanimpacientes.wordpress.com/

https://www.facebook.com/SaluDesenchufada

http://www.lessismoremedicine.com/

- *Up-To-Date*: Subscription-based online "text-book" of medicine with continuing medical education, podcasts, calculators, and patient education resources that isn't 100 percent industry-free but strives to come as close as possible (USA)

  http://www.uptodate.com/home

- *VNS Message Board*: Extensive information about the VNS device; Dennis Fegan and Donna Baum post here, along with many others (USA)

  http://www.vnsmessageboard.com/

- *Woody Matters*: Focuses on the harm caused by antidepressants (USA)

  www.woodymatters.com

RESOURCES FOR JOURNALISTS

- *Health News Review*: Provides the best critical analyses available of media health news reporting (USA)

  https://www.healthnewsreview.org/

- *The List*: An international list of industry-independent experts for the media, guidelines panels, and regulatory agencies (USA). Updated list available at:

  https://www.jeannelenzer.com/

  and

  https://www.healthnewsreview.org/

Acknowledgments

I'm deeply indebted to many more people than those whose names appear in this book. However, I'd like to start by thanking Annabel Ferriman, my former editor, who gave me my first break, assigning me to write an investigative piece for *The BMJ*.

Many years ago, I told Jerry Hoffman that I wanted to write a "biography of his ideas." He has an enthusiastic following of medical students and doctors who appreciate his incisive analyses of medical research and his decades-long and consistent stance against accepting industry blandishments. While Jerry declined to comment on certain subjects addressed in this book, his influence on my thinking is profound, and virtually all the concepts, analyses, and viewpoints in this book have been in some way touched or influenced by Jerry. Of course, any mistakes are my own.

Shannon Brownlee, my writing partner, dearest friend, colleague, and sparring partner, has not only taught me a good deal about writing but has also taught me how to argue with love. She has been a shining light. Without her, this book would not have been possible.

This book bears the imprint of several medical giants whose time, interviews, and writings have also shaped this book: John Ioannidis, who has repeatedly demonstrated the messiness of medical research and its many distortions; the inimitable Bernard Lown and his colleague Vikas Saini, who both live by Bernard's creed—"Do as much *for* patients and as little as possible *to* patients"; Marcia Angell, whose commitment to disentangling money and medicine has inspired me and many others; and Richard Smith and Fiona Godlee, who as editors in chief of *The BMJ* set a high bar for medical journals and my own work.

For a better understanding of the FDA, its approval process, oversight in general, and the VNS device in particular, I am grateful to Ronald Kavanagh, Paul Thacker, Diana Zuckerman, Sidney Wolfe, Michael Carome, Marc-André Gagnon, Larry Kessler, Suzanne Parisian, Madris Tomes, and Deborah Zarin. I'd also like to thank several experts who asked not to be named for fear of losing their jobs.

Experts who expanded my understanding of scientific biases, financial conflicts of interest, and institutional corruption include: Joel Lexchin, Jerome Kassirer, Alan Cassels, John Abramson, Vinay Prasad, Peter Goetzsche, Rita Redberg, Otis Brawley, Kenneth Lin, Sheldon Krimsky, Neil Calman, Michael Wilkes, Deb Cohen, Steven Nissen, Adriane Fugh-Berman, Roy Poses, Barnett Kramer, Carl Heneghan, Lisa Bero, Nortin Hadler, Mohammad Zakaria Pezeshki, Steven Woloshin, Gil Welch, Lisa Schwartz, David Himmelstein, Steffie Woolhandler, Howard Brody, and Linda Marsa.

For explanations regarding the problems and possibilities of healthcare delivery, I'm indebted to Wendell Potter, T. R. Reid, John Geyman, and Physicians for a National Health Program. For an inspirational view of what independent research can do, I'm indebted to Donald Light and Antonio Maturo, authors of *Good Pharma*, and the Mario Negri Institute. I'm also indebted to the many patients who educated me about their experiences with implants, from surgical mesh to certain birth-control implants, whose stories I wasn't able to include. Their experiences drove me to persist with a "big picture" depiction of the problems, which I hope will in some small way help lead to solutions for this vastly underregulated industry.

The Knight Science Journalism Fellowship and many of my fellow journalists around the globe, especially Gary Schwitzer and the folks at *HealthNewsReview,* have inspired me, humbled me, and kept me kicking for the many years it took me to write this book—to them and to the Birdies, I am forever grateful.

Thanks to Margaret Cirillo and Mary Evans, who with expert speed kept me supplied with medical articles I requested.

To my agent, Eileen Cope: you're the best cheerleader a writer could ask for. To Karl Weber, a consulting editor who tore my first manuscript apart and made me write a better book, thank you for your vision and kindness. To Jean Garnet, my editor at Little, Brown, thanks for expecting better after the first submission. To my publisher, I can only thank Eileen for ensuring that I signed with you—she couldn't have chosen more wisely.

To Dennis Fegan and his family: you were incredibly kind to let me into your homes and lives. Your willingness to share your memories and insights with a stranger, and now the world, is a testament to the humor and strength I observed in your family. Dennis, you kept at it. You persevered. And even when all remedies for you were long gone, you kept working and researching with only the hope that you might help others. You are a star.

And as is so often the case, writing a book can be all-consuming. Not only did my family allow me to pursue this work, but the wisdom and kindness of my husband, John Calhoun, also helped me see shades of gray where I often saw only black and white. Special thanks to my son, Mahtik "Tiki" Calhoun, who was so understanding throughout, and to my wonderful muse, Ada Prior.

Notes

1. Goodman SL, Geiderman JM, Bernstein IJ. Prophylactic lidocaine in suspected acute myocardial infarction. *JACEP.* 1979;8(6):221–224. http://www.ncbi.nlm.nih.gov/pubmed/449144.

2. Pigman E, Smith M. Prehospital prophylactic lidocaine for uncomplicated acute myocardial infarction [editorial; comment]. *J Emerg Med.* 1993;11(6):753–755. http://www.ncbi.nlm.nih.gov/pubmed/8157915.

3. Pratt CM, Moye LA. The cardiac arrhythmia suppression trial: casting suppression in a different light. *Circulation.* 1995;91(1):245–247. http://circ.ahajournals.org/content/91/1/245.full.

4. Newman TB. A black-box warning for antidepressants in children? *N Engl J Med.* 2004;351(16):1595–1598. PM:15483275.

5. Waxman H. The marketing of Vioxx to physicians. https://democrats-oversight.house.gov/sites/democrats.oversight.house.gov/files/documents/20050505114932-41272.pdf. 2005.

6. Bernadette T. Firm misled doctors on Vioxx, panel says sales staff told not to discuss risk study. *San Francisco Chronicle* 2005. http://www.sfgate.com/cgi-bin/article.cgi?file=/c/a/2005/05/06/VIOXX.TMP.

7. Suz R. Journal: drug sales based on "seriously biased" data: Celebrex, Vioxx cited for problems, claims. *Washington Post* 2002: HE01.

8. Lenzer J. US government agency to investigate FDA over rofecoxib. *BMJ.* 2004;329(7472):935. http://bmj.bmjjournals.com/cgi/content/full/329/7472/935.

9. Home PD, Pocock SJ, Beck-Nielsen H, et al. Rosiglitazone evaluated for cardiovascular outcomes in oral agent combination therapy for type 2 diabetes (RECORD): a multicentre, randomised, open-label trial. *Lancet.* Jun 20, 2009, 2009;373(9681):2125–2135. http://dx.doi.org/10.1016/S0140-6736(09)60953-3.

10. Nissen SE, Wolski K. Effect of Rosiglitazone on the risk of myocardial infarction and death from cardiovascular causes. *N Engl J Med.* 2007;356(24):2457–2471. http://content.nejm.org/cgi/content/abstract/356/24/2457.

11. Rosen CJ. The rosiglitazone story—lessons from an FDA advisory committee meeting. *N Engl J Med.* 2007;357(9):844–846. http://www.nejm.org/doi/full/10.1056/NEJMp078167.

12. Crosse M. Medical Devices: FDA Should Take Steps to Ensure That High-Risk Device Types Are Approved through the Most Stringent Premarket Review Process. United States Government Accountability Office; January 2009. www.gao.gov/assets/290/284882.pdf.

13. Rome BN, Kramer DB, Kesselheim AS. FDA approval of cardiac implantable electronic devices via original and supplement premarket approval pathways, 1979–2012. *JAMA.* 2014;311(4):385–391. http://dx.doi.org/10.1001/jama.2013.284986.

14. Johnson JA. FDA Regulation of Medical Devices. Congressional Research Service; Sept 14, 2016. https://fas.org/sgp/crs/misc/R42130.pdf.

15. Dhruva SS, Bero LA, Redberg RF. Strength of study evidence examined by the FDA in premarket approval of cardiovascular devices. *JAMA.* 2009;302(24):2679–2685. http://jama.jamanetwork.com/article.aspx?articleid=185124.

16. Braunwald E. A conversation with Eugene Braunwald. Interview by Ushma S. Neill. *J Clin Invest.* Jan 2, 2013;123(1):1–2. http://www.ncbi.nlm.nih.gov/pubmed/23281402 and https://www.youtube.com/watch?v=Z19mCY-Rb2A.

17. Lee TH. *Eugene Braunwald and the Rise of Modern Medicine.* Cambridge, MA: Harvard University Press; 2013.

18. Luderitz B. Bernard Lown. *J Interv Card Electrophysiol.* Jun, 2004;10(3):293–294. https://www.ncbi.nlm.nih.gov/pubmed/15133370.

19. Maddocks I. Bernard Lown and 21 years of International Physicians for Prevention of Nuclear War. *Med Confl Surviv.* Jan–Mar, 2003;19(1):1–3. https://www.ncbi.nlm.nih.gov/pubmed/12776930.

20. Banerjee A. Bernard Lown: the nonagenarian blogger with a lifelong thirst for combining clinical practice and social responsibility. *Eur Heart J.* May, 2013;34(18):1316–1317. https://www.ncbi.nlm.nih.gov/pubmed/23802251.

21. Lown B, Amarasingham R, Neuman J. New method for terminating cardiac arrhythmias: use of synchronized capacitor discharge. *JAMA.* Aug 1, 1986;256(5):621–627. https://www.ncbi.nlm.nih.gov/pubmed/3522950.

22. Eisenberg M. The resuscitation greats. Bernard Lown and defibrillation. *Resuscitation.* May, 2006;69(2):171–173. https://www.ncbi.nlm.nih.gov/pubmed/16650729.

23. Todd KH, Lee T, Hoffman JR. The effect of ethnicity on physician estimates of pain severity in patients with isolated extremity trauma. *JAMA.* 1994;271(12):925–928.

24. Miura BR, Schreiger DL, Hoffman JR. What an ED doc will do for a buck: implications for survey research. *Ann Emerg Med.* Nov, 1997;30(5):713–714. http://www.ncbi.nlm.nih.gov/pubmed/9360591.

25. Hoffman JR, Cooper RJ. Stroke thrombolysis: we need new data, not more reviews. *Lancet Neurol.* Apr, 2005;4(4):204–205. http://www.ncbi.nlm.nih.gov/pubmed/15778096.

26. Bell DS, Hays RD, Hoffman JR, Day FC, Higa JK, Wilkes MS. A test of knowledge about prostate cancer screening. Online pilot evaluation among Southern California Physicians. *J Gen Intern Med.* Apr, 2006;21(4):310–314. http://www.ncbi.nlm.nih.gov/pubmed/16499545.

27. Hoffman JR, Cooper RJ. Overdiagnosis of disease: a modern epidemic. *Arch Intern Med.* 2012;172(15):1123–1124. http://dx.doi.org/10.1001/archinternmed.2012.3319.

28. Kanzaria HK, Hoffman JR, Probst MA, Caloyeras JP, Berry SH, Brook RH. Emergency physician perceptions of medically unnecessary advanced diagnostic imaging. *Acad Emerg Med.* Apr, 2015;22(4):390–398.

29. Mackenbach JP. Politics is nothing but medicine at a larger scale: reflections on public health's biggest idea. *J Epidemiol Community Health.* Mar, 2009;63(3):181–184.

30. Woolf SH, Aron L. *US Health in International Perspective: Shorter Lives, Poorer Health*: Washington, DC: National Academies Press; 2013.

31. U.S. Health Care from a Global Perspective. Commonwealth Fund; 2015. http://www.commonwealthfund.org/publications/issue-briefs/2015/oct/us-health-care-from-a-global-perspective.

32. World Population Prospects. Volume 1: Comprehensive Tables. 2015 revision. United Nations Department of Economic and Social Affairs; 2015. https://esa.un.org/unpd/wpp/Publications/Files/WPP2015_Volume-I_Comprehensive-Tables.pdf.

33. Mortality in the United States, 2015. Centers for Disease Control and Prevention: National Center for Health Statistics; 2015. https://www.cdc.gov/nchs/products/databriefs/db267.htm.

34. Khazan O. Why American women aren't living as long as they should. *The Atlantic* 2014. http://www.theatlantic.com/health/archive/2014/01/why-american-women-arent-living-as-long-as-they-should/282984/.

35. Kindig DA, Cheng ER. Even as mortality fell in most US counties, female mortality nonetheless rose in 42.8 percent of counties from 1992 to 2006. *Health Aff.* 2013;32(3):451–458. http://content.healthaffairs.org/content/32/3/451.abstract.

36. Olshansky SJ, Antonucci T, Berkman L, et al. Differences in life expectancy due to race and educational differences are widening, and many may not catch up. *Health Aff.* 2012;31(8):1803–1813. http://content.healthaffairs.org/content/31/8/1803.abstract.

37. Organisation for Economic Co-operation and Development. Daily Smokers. 2014. https://data.oecd.org/healthrisk/daily-smokers.htm#indicator-chart.

38. Organisation for Economic Co-operation and Development. Alcohol Consumption. 2014. https://data.oecd.org/healthrisk/alcohol-consumption.htm.

39. Berwick DM, Hackbarth AD. Eliminating waste in US health care. *JAMA.* Apr 11, 2012;307(14):1513–1516. https://www.ncbi.nlm.nih.gov/pubmed/22419800.

40. Ferguson TB, Jr. The Institute of Medicine committee report "best care at lower cost: the path to continuously learning health care." *Circ Cardiovasc Qual Outcomes.* Nov, 2012;5(6):e93–94. https://www.ncbi.nlm.nih.gov/pubmed/23170008.

41. *Health Affairs.* Health Policy Brief: Reducing Waste in Health Care. Dec 13, 2012. http://healthaffairs.org/healthpolicybriefs/brief_pdfs/healthpolicybrief_82.pdf.

42. Allen M. How many die from medical mistakes in U.S. hospitals? *ProPublica* 2013. https://www.propublica.org/article/how-many-die-from-medical-mistakes-in-us-hospitals.

43. Moore TJ, Furberg CD, Cohen MR. Anticoagulants the Leading Reported Drug Risk in 2011. *QuarterWatch: Monitoring FDA MedWatch Reports.* Institute for Safe Medication Practices2012. http://www.omsj.org/reports/2011Q4.pdf.

44. Wilper AP, Woolhandler S, Lasser KE, McCormick D, Bor DH, Himmelstein DU. Health insurance and mortality in US adults. *Am J Public Health.* Dec, 2009;99(12):2289–2295. http://www.ncbi.nlm.nih.gov/pubmed/19762659.

45. Himmelstein DU, Thorne D, Warren E, Woolhandler S. Medical bankruptcy in the United States, 2007: results of a national study. *Am J Med.* Aug, 2009;122(8):741–746. http://www.ncbi.nlm.nih.gov/pubmed/19501347.

46. Woolhandler S, Himmelstein DU. Grim prognosis for Massachusetts reform. *Health Aff.* Mar–Apr, 2009;28(2):604–605; author reply 605. http://www.ncbi.nlm.nih.gov/pubmed/19276039.

47. Himmelstein DU, Thorne D, Woolhandler S. Medical bankruptcy in Massachusetts: has health reform made a difference? *Am J Med.* Mar, 2011;124(3):224–228. http://www.ncbi.nlm.nih.gov/pubmed/21396505.

48. Kawachi I, Kennedy BP. Health and social cohesion: why care about income inequality? *BMJ.* 1997;314(7086):1037.

49. Marmot M, Ryff CD, Bumpass LL, Shipley M, Marks NF. Social inequalities in health: next questions and converging evidence. *Soc Sci Med.* 1997;44(6):901–910.

50. Pappas G, Queen S, Hadden W, Fisher G. The increasing disparity in mortality between socioeconomic groups in the United States, 1960 and 1986. *N Engl J Med.* 1993;329(2):103–109.

51. Kawachi I, Kennedy BP, Lochner K, Prothrow-Stith D. Social capital, income inequality, and mortality. *Am J Public Health.* 1997;87(9):1491–1498.

52. Johnston DC. The true cost of national security: the Pentagon and the White House focus on the core defense budget, but that's not the half of it. *Columbia Journalism Review* 2013. http://www.cjr.org/united_states_project/the_true_cost_of_national_secu.php.

53. Kaiser Health Tracker. 2016. http://www.healthsystemtracker.org/interactive/?display=U.S.%2520%2524%2520Billions&service=All%2520Types%2520of%2520Services.

54. Stern AM, Markel H. The history of vaccines and immunization: familiar patterns, new challenges. *Health Aff.* 2005;24(3):611–621. http://content.healthaffairs.org/content/24/3/611.abstract.

55. Impactscan.org. A brief history of the CT. http://www.impactscan.org/CThistory.htm.

56. Cools J. Improvements in the survival of children and adolescents with acute lymphoblastic leukemia. *Haematologica.* 2012;97(5):635-635. http://www.ncbi.nlm.nih.gov/pmc/articles/PMC3342961/.

57. Forkus B. Ear on a mouse. http://openwetware.org/wiki/Ear_on_a_Mouse,_by_Brittany_Forkus.

58. Lenzer J. Have we entered the stem cell era? *Discover* 2009. http://discovermagazine.com/2009/nov/14-have-we-entered-the-stem-cell-era.

59. American Academy of Anti-Aging Medicine. http://www.a4m.com/.

60. Jenkins HW, Jr. Will Google's Ray Kurzweil live forever? *Wall Street Journal* 2013. http://www.wsj.com/articles/SB10001424127887324504704578412581386515510.

61. Transparency International asks health care professionals about health care corruption. 2016. http://hcrenewal.blogspot.com/search/label/health%20care%20corruption.

62. Schneider A, Geewax M. On-the-job deaths spiking as oil drilling quickly expands. *All Things Considered.* 2013. http://www.npr.org/2013/12/27/250807226/on-the-job-deaths-spiking-as-oil-drilling-quickly-expands.

63. Adams SM, Knowles PD. Evaluation of a first seizure. *Am Fam Physician.* May 1, 2007;75(9):1342–1347.

64. Holmes G, Sirven J, Fisher RS. Temporal lobe epilepsy. http://www.epilepsy.com/learn/types-epilepsy-syndromes/temporal-lobe-epilepsy.

65. Laxer KD, Trinka E, Hirsch LJ, et al. The consequences of refractory epilepsy and its treatment. *Epilepsy Behav.* Aug, 2014;37:59–70. http://www.ncbi.nlm.nih.gov/pubmed/24980390.

66. French JA. Refractory epilepsy: clinical overview. *Epilepsia.* 2007;48 Suppl 1:3–7.

67. Restak R. Complex partial seizures present diagnostic challenge. *Psychiatric Times* 1995. www.psychiatrictimes.com/articles/complex-partial-seizures-present-diagnostic-challenge.

68. Mirsattari SM, Gofton TE, Chong DJ. Misdiagnosis of epileptic seizures as manifestations of psychiatric illnesses. *Can J Neurol Sci.* May, 2011;38(3):487–493.

69. Packer L, Tritschler HJ, Wessel K. Neuroprotection by the metabolic antioxidant alpha-lipoic acid. *Free Radic Biol Med.* 1997;22(1–2):359-378. PM:0008958163.

70. Braunwald E. Adventures in cardiovascular research. *Circulation.* Jul 14, 2009;120(2):170–180. http://www.ncbi.nlm.nih.gov/pubmed/19597062.

71. Lydon C. The rise of modern medicine. *Radio Open Source.* 2014. http://radioopensource.org/rise-modern-medicine/.

72. Forrester JS, Harold JG. Eugene Braunwald, MD, MACC, a lifetime of achievements and a legend of cardiology. *Cardiology* 2014. http://www.acc.org/latest-in-cardiology/articles/2014/02/27/13/20/eugene-braunwald-md-macc-a-lifetime-of-achievements-and-a-legend-of-cardiology.

73. Braunwald E, Sabatine MS. The Thrombolysis in Myocardial Infarction (TIMI) Study Group experience. *J Thorac Cardiovasc Surg.* 2012;144(4):762–770. doi: 710.1016/j.jtcvs.2012.1007.1001. Epub 2012 Aug 1015.

74. Sabatine MS. What is the TIMI Study Group? In: Institute of Medicine. *Implementing a National Cancer Clinical Trials System for the 21st Century.* Washington, DC: National Academies Press; 2013.

75. Stoney WS. Evolution of cardiopulmonary bypass. *Circulation.* 2009;119(21):2844–2853. http://circ.ahajournals.org/content/119/21/2844.short.

76. Morrow AG, Braunwald E. Functional aortic stenosis; a malformation characterized by resistance to left ventricular outflow without anatomic obstruction. *Circulation.* Aug, 1959;20(2):181–189. http://www.ncbi.nlm.nih.gov/pubmed/13671704.

77. Fegan D. VNS: A Cure All??? 2011. http://www.vnsmessageboard.com/index.php?topic=3933.0;all.

78. Epilepsy Foundation. Atonic and tonic seizures. http://www.epilepsy.com/learn/treating-seizures-and-epilepsy/first-aid/atonic-and-tonic-seizures.

79. Interview with Larry Johnson (in person), January 11, 2014.

80. Nickels KC, Grossardt BR, Wirrell EC. Epilepsy-related mortality is low in children: a 30 year population-based study in Olmsted County, MN. *Epilepsia.* 2012;53(12):2164–2171. http://www.ncbi.nlm.nih.gov/pmc/articles/PMC3766953/.

81. Tomson T, Walczak T, Sillanpaa M, Sander JW. Sudden unexpected death in epilepsy: a review of incidence and risk factors. *Epilepsia.* 2005;46 Suppl 11:54–61. http://www.ncbi.nlm.nih.gov/pubmed/16393182.

82. Spencer DC. SUDEP: sudden unexpected death in epilepsy on placebo? *Epilepsy Currents.* 2012;12(2):51–52. http://www.ncbi.nlm.nih.gov/pubmed/22473539.

83. Velagapudi P, Turagam M, Laurence T, Kocheril A. Cardiac arrhythmias and sudden unexpected death in epilepsy (SUDEP). *Pacing Clin Electrophysiol.* 2012;35(3):363–370. http://www.ncbi.nlm.nih.gov/pubmed/22126214.

84. Ludmerer KM. Health care. In: Kutler SI, ed. *Dictionary of American History.* Vol 4. 3rd ed. New York: Charles Scribner's Sons; 2003:115–118.

85. Preskitt JT. Health care reimbursement: Clemens to Clinton. *Baylor University Medical Center Proceedings.* 2008;21(1):40–44. http://www.ncbi.nlm.nih.gov/pmc/articles/PMC2190551/.

86. Thomasson M. Health insurance in the United States. https://eh.net/encyclopedia/health-insurance-in-the-united-states/, 2016.

87. Kernahan PJ. Was there ever a "golden age" of medicine? *Minn Med.* 2012;95(9):41–45. http://pubs.royle.com/display_article.php?id=1159666.

88. Stevens RA. Health care in the early 1960s. *Health Care Financ Rev.* 1996;18(2):11–22. http://www.ssa.gov/history/pdf/HealthCareEarly1960s.pdf.

89. Medicine: doctors' pay. *Time* 1951. http://content.time.com/time/magazine/article/0,9171,815193,00.html.

90. Brownlee S. *Overtreated: Why Too Much Medicine Is Making Us Sicker and Poorer.* New York: Bloomsbury USA; 2007.

91. Starr P. *The Social Transformation of Medicine: The Rise of a Sovereign Profession and the Making of a Vast Industry.* New York: Basic Books; 1982.

92. Levit KR, Olin GL, Letsch SW. Americans' health insurance coverage, 1980–91. *Health Care Financ Rev.* 1992;14(1):31–57. http://www.ncbi.nlm.nih.gov/pmc/articles/PMC4193314/.

93. Herman B. 12 Statistics on CT Scanner Costs. *Becker's Hospital Review* 2012. http://www.beckershospitalreview.com/hospital-key-specialties/12-statistics-on-ct-scanner-costs.html.

94. Brody H. *Hooked: Ethics, the Medical Profession, and the Pharmaceutical Industry.* Lanham, MD: Rowman & Littlefield; 2007.

95. National health expenditures data 1960–2014. Centers for Medicare and Medicaid Services. 2014. https://www.cms.gov/Research-Statistics-Data-and-Systems/Statistics-Trends-and-Reports/NationalHealthExpendData/Downloads/NHEGDP14.zip.

96. Government Accountability Office. Medical Device Companies: Trends in Reported Net Sales and Profits Before and After Implementation of the Patient Protection and Affordable Care Act. 6/30/2015. http://www.gao.gov/assets/680/671094.pdf.

97. Meier B. Costs surge for medical devices, but benefits are opaque. *New York Times* 2009. http://www.nytimes.com/2009/11/05/business/05device.html?_r=0.

98. Swirsky L. Health policy brief: medical device manufacturer profits. Consumers Union. 2013. http://consumersunion.org/research/health-policy-brief-medical-device-manufacturer-profits/.

99. US Food and Drug Administration. UDI basics. 2015. http://www.fda.gov/MedicalDevices/DeviceRegulationandGuidance/UniqueDeviceIdentification/UDIBasics/default.htm.

100. Lenzer J, Brownlee S. Why the FDA can't protect the public. *BMJ.* 2010;341:c4753. http://www.bmj.com/content/341/bmj.c4753.long.

101. Daniel G, Colvin H, Khaterzai S, McClellan M, Pranav A. *Strengthening Patient Care: Building an Effective National Medical Device Surveillance System.* Washington, DC: Brookings Institution; 2015. http://www.brookings.edu/research/papers/2015/02/23-medical-device-postmarket-surveillance-roadmap-daniel.

102. Chelimsky E. Medical Devices: Early Warning of Problems Is Hampered by Severe Underreporting. Government Accountability Office.1986. http://www.gao.gov/products/PEMD-87-1.

103. Zuckerman DM, Brown P, Nissen SE. Medical device recalls and the FDA approval process. *Arch Intern Med.* 2011;171(11):1006–1011. http://dx.doi.org/10.1001/archinternmed.2011.30.

104. Gholipour B. New implant no longer dangerous in MRI. *LiveScience* 2013. http://www.livescience.com/38926-new-mri-safe-implant.html.

105. 3-Tesla MR safety information for implants and devices. MRISafety.com. 2017. http://www.mrisafety.com/SafetyInfov.asp?SafetyInfoID=227.

106. Hoshaw L. Millions of Americans use medical devices that may be vulnerable to hacking. KQED News. 2015. https://ww2.kqed.org/futureofyou/2015/08/03/millions-of-americans-use-medical-devices-that-are-vulnerable-to-hacking/.

107. Cleary D. Could a wireless pacemaker let hackers take control of your life? *Science* 2015. http://www.sciencemag.org/news/2015/02/could-wireless-pacemaker-let-hackers-take-control-your-heart.

108. Kirk J. Pacemaker hack can deliver deadly 830-volt jolt. *ComputerWorld* 2012. http://www.computerworld.com/article/2492453/malware-vulnerabilities/pacemaker-hack-can-deliver-deadly-830-volt-jolt.html.

109. Hacker dies days before he was to reveal how to remotely kill pacemaker patients. RT. 2013. https://www.rt.com/usa/hacker-pacemaker-barnaby-jack-639/.

110. Newman L. Medical devices are the next security nightmare. *Wired* 2017. https://www.wired.com/2017/03/medical-devices-next-security-nightmare/.

111. Memorandum of Understanding Between the Centers for Medicare and Medicaid Services Coverage and Analysis Group and the U.S. Food and Drug Administration Center for Devices and Radiological Health Regarding Categorization of Investigational Devices. Mou 225-16-024. 2016. http://www.fda.gov/AboutFDA/PartnershipsCollaborations/MemorandaofUnderstandingMOUs/DomesticMOUs/ucm477091.htm.

112. Talbot D. Computer viruses are "rampant" on medical devices in hospitals. *MIT Technology Review.* Oct 17, 2012. https://www.technologyreview.com/s/429616/computer-viruses-are-rampant-on-medical-devices-in-hospitals/.

113. Poole JE, Gleva MJ, Mela T, et al. Complication rates associated with pacemaker or implantable cardioverter-defibrillator generator replacements and upgrade procedures: results from the REPLACE registry. *Circulation.* 2010;122(16):1553–1561. https://www.ncbi.nlm.nih.gov/pubmed/20921437.

114. Letter from Juan E. Bahamon, MD, to Dennis Fegan dated Dec 12, 2006.

115. Braunwald E, Epstein SE, Glick G, Wechsler AS, Braunwald NS. Relief of angina pectoris by electrical stimulation of the carotid-sinus nerves. *N Engl J Med.* 1967;277(24):1278–1283. http://www.nejm.org/doi/full/10.1056/NEJM196712142772402.

116. Braunwald E, Vatner SF, Braunwald NS, Sobel BE. Carotid sinus nerve stimulation in the treatment of angina pectoris and supraventricular tachycardia. *West J Med.* 1970;112(3):41–50.

117. Langreth R. Rewiring the brain. *Forbes* 2001. http://www.forbes.com/forbes/2001/0305/160.html.

118. Infitialis. Under surveillance: blowing the whistle on Cyberonics. *StreetSweeper* 2013. http://www.thestreetsweeper.org/undersurveillance/Blowing_the_Whistle_on_Cyberonics.

119. Medical Device and Diagostic Industry. The two-year turnaround. 2008. http://www.mddionline.com/article/two-year-turnaround.

120. Mabin DC. BMJ should declare its own conflict of interest. *BMJ.* 1995;311(7009):878–879. PM:0007580526.

121. Phone interview with Robert "Skip" Cummins, April 2, 2015.

122. Nocera J. A C.E.O. who carries a big stick. *New York Times* 2005. http://query.nytimes.com/gst/fullpage.html?res=9407EFDD1F30F93BA35753C1A9639C8B63=.

123. Hines JZ, Lurie P, Yu E, Wolfe S. Left to their own devices: breakdowns in United States medical device premarket review. *PLoS Med.* 2010;7(7):e1000280. http://www.ncbi.nlm.nih.gov/pmc/articles/PMC2903853/.

124. Chan PS, Patel MR, Klein LW, et al. Appropriateness of percutaneous coronary intervention. *JAMA.* 2011;306(1):53–61. http://www.ncbi.nlm.nih.gov/pubmed/21730241.

125. Rothberg MB, Scherer L, Kashef M, et al. The effect of information presentation on beliefs about the benefits of elective percutaneous coronary intervention. *JAMA Intern Med.* 2014;174(10):1623–1629. http://dx.doi.org/10.1001/jamainternmed.2014.3331.

126. Rothberg MB, Sivalingam SK, Ashraf J, et al. Patients' and cardiologists' perceptions of the benefits of percutaneous coronary intervention for stable coronary disease. *Ann Intern Med.* 2010;153(5):307–313. http://www.ncbi.nlm.nih.gov/pubmed/20820040.

127. Bradley SM, Spertus JA, Kennedy KF, et al. Patient selection for diagnostic coronary

angiography and hospital-level percutaneous coronary intervention appropriateness: insights from the national cardiovascular data registry. *JAMA Intern Med.* 2014;174 (10):1630–1639. http://dx.doi.org/10.1001/jamainternmed.2014.3904.

128. Brown DL, Redberg RF. Continuing use of prophylactic percutaneous coronary intervention in patients with stable coronary artery disease despite evidence of no benefit: déjà vu all over again. *JAMA Intern Med.* May 1, 2016;176(5):597–598. http://www.ncbi.nlm.nih.gov/pubmed/27019878.

129. Lin GA, Dudley RA, Redberg RF. Cardiologists' use of percutaneous coronary interventions for stable coronary artery disease. *Arch Intern Med.* 2007;167(15):1604–1609.

130. Stergiopoulos K, Brown DL. Initial coronary stent implantation with medical therapy vs medical therapy alone for stable coronary artery disease: meta-analysis of randomized controlled trials. *Arch Intern Med.* 2012;172(4):312–319. http://www.ncbi.nlm.nih.gov/pubmed/22371919.

131. Boden WE, O'Rourke RA, Teo KK, et al. Optimal medical therapy with or without PCI for stable coronary disease. *N Engl J Med.* 2007;356(15):1503–1516. http://www.nejm.org/doi/full/10.1056/NEJMoa070829.

132. Interview with Rita Redberg (phone and e-mail), May 7, 2017.

133. Tenth meeting of FDA's Center for Devices and Radiological Health Neurological Devices Panel. 1997. www.fda.gov/ohrms/dockets/ac/97/transcpt/3299t1.pdf.

134. Jones D. Company news: St. Jude Medical to buy maker of neurology devices. *New York Times* 1996. http://www.nytimes.com/1996/04/09/business/company-news-st-jude-medical-to-buy-maker-of-neurology-devices.html.

135. Handforth A, DeGiorgio CM, Schachter SC, et al. Vagus nerve stimulation therapy for partial-onset seizures: a randomized active-control trial. *Neurology.* 1998;51(1):48–55. http://www.neurology.org/cgi/content/abstract/51/1/48.

136. Lurie P, Stine N, Wolfe S (Public Citizen). Petition to reverse the FDA's prior approval of the vagus nerve stimulation (VNS) device for the management of treatment-resistant depression. 2006. http://www.fda.gov/ohrms/dockets/dockets/06p0370/06p-0370-cp00001-vol1.pdf.

137. Malisow C. Exposed nerve. *Houston Press* 2005. http://www.houstonpress.com/2005-04-07/news/exposed-nerve/.

138. Center for Responsive Politics. Annual lobbying by Cyberonics Inc. https://www.opensecrets.org/lobby/clientsum.php?id=D000049935&year=2015. Accessed August 15, 2016.

139. Smith EB. Special report: Insiders made nearly $50M trading a money-losing company's stock. *USA Today* 2006. http://usatoday30.usatoday.com/money/companies/management/2006-11-20-cyberonics-usat_x.htm.

140. Is Tony Coelho a crook? *Slate* 2000. http://www.slate.com/articles/news_and_politics/explainer/2000/04/is_tony_coelho_a_crook.html.

141. Union of Concerned Scientists. FDA medical device approval based on politics, not science. 2009. http://www.ucsusa.org/our-work/center-science-and-democracy/promoting-scientific-integrity/fda-medical-device-approval.html#.V4apZzWi4ZE.

142. Nakashima E, Rein L. FDA staffers sue agency over surveillance of personal e-mail. *Washington Post* 2012. https://www.washingtonpost.com/world/national-security/fda-staffers-sue-agency-over-surveillance-of-personal-e-mail/2012/01/23/gIQAj34DbQ_story.html.

143. Feder BJ. Head of Cyberonics resigns as options inquiry expands. *New York Times* 2006. http://www.nytimes.com/2006/11/21/business/21device.html?dlbk.

144. VNS message board. http://www.vnsmessageboard.com/.

145. Iriarte J, Urrestarazu E, Alegre M, et al. Late-onset periodic asystolia during vagus nerve stimulation. *Epilepsia.* 2009;50(4):928–932. https://www.ncbi.nlm.nih.gov/pubmed/19055490.

146. Bryan Olin. E-mail from Cyberonics to *The BMJ.* March 15, 2010.

147. Junod SW. FDA and clinical drug trials: a short history. 2016. http://www.fda.gov/AboutFDA/WhatWeDo/History/Overviews/ucm304485.htm.

148. Lex JR, Jr. Dr. Joseph Rohan Lex, Jr., MD, FAAEM: the physician-pharmaceutical industry relationship. *J Law Health.* 2004;18(2):323. http://engagedscholarship.csuohio.edu/cgi/viewcontent.cgi?article=1126&context=jlh.

149. Mann H, Djulbegovic B. Comparator bias: why comparisons must address genuine uncertainties. *JLL Bulletin: Commentaries on the history of treatment evaluation.* 2012. http://www.jameslindlibrary.org/articles/comparator-bias-why-comparisons-must-address-genuine-uncertainties/.

150. Hoffmann TC, Del Mar C. Patients' expectations of the benefits and harms of treatments, screening, and tests: a systematic review. *JAMA Intern Med.* 2015;175(2):274–286. http://dx.doi.org/10.1001/jamainternmed.2014.6016.

151. Hoffmann TC, Del Mar C. Clinicians' expectations of the benefits and harms of treatments, screening, and tests: a systematic review. *JAMA Intern Med.* 2017;177(3):407–419. http://dx.doi.org/10.1001/jamainternmed.2016.8254.

152. Lenzer J. Why aren't the US Centers for Disease Control and Food and Drug Administration speaking with one voice on flu? *BMJ.* 2015-02-05 14:40:22, 2015;350. http://www.bmj.com/content/350/bmj.h658.

153. Jefferson T, Jones M, Doshi P, Del Mar C. Neuraminidase inhibitors for preventing and treating influenza in healthy adults: systematic review and meta-analysis. *BMJ.* 2009;339(dec07_2):b5106. http://www.bmj.com/cgi/content/abstract/339/dec07_2/b5106.

154. Ioannidis JP. Why most published research findings are false. *PLoS Med.* 2005;2(8):e124. http://journals.plos.org/plosmedicine/article?id=10.1371/journal.pmed.0020124.

155. Ioannidis JP. Contradicted and initially stronger effects in highly cited clinical research. *JAMA* 2005;294(2):218–228. http://jamanetwork.com/journals/jama/fullarticle/2012.

156. Heres S, Davis J, Maino K, Jetzinger E, Kissling W, Leucht S. Why olanzapine beats risperidone, risperidone beats quetiapine, and quetiapine beats olanzapine: an exploratory analysis of head-to-head comparison studies of second-generation antipsychotics. *Am J Psychiatry.* 2006;163(2):185–194. PM:16449469.

157. Brownlee S, Lenzer J. The problem with medicine: we don't know if most of it works. *Discover* 2010. http://discovermagazine.com/2010/nov/11-the-problem-with-medicine-dont-know-if-most-works.

158. MAUDE: Manufacturer and User Facility Device Experience. https://www.accessdata.fda.gov/scripts/cdrh/cfdocs/cfmaude/TextSearch.cfm.

159. Phone interview with Diana Zuckerman, May 21, 2016.

160. Phone interview with Mark Bruley, May 14, 2009.

161. Cyberonics. Issue report [into Dennis Fegan's case]. Released under the FOIA from the State of Texas Department of Health investigation 8/25/2009.

162. Armstrong R, Parnis S, Scott T, inventors; Google Patents, assignee. Providing multiple signal modes for a medical device. 2007. https://encrypted.google.com/patents/US20070100377.

163. Barrett B, Parnis S, Maschino S, Guzman A, inventors; Google Patents, assignee. Cranial nerve stimulation to treat a hearing disorder. 2007. http://www.google.com.gi/patents/US20070027504.

164. Inman D, Parnis S, Guzman A, inventors; Google Patents, assignee. Method and apparatus for forming insulated implantable electrodes. 2007. https://www.google.com/patents/US20070255320.

165. Maschino S, Parnis S, Armstrong S, inventors; Google Patents, assignee. Identification of electrodes for nerve stimulation in the treatment of eating disorders. 2006. https://www.google.com/patents/US7310557.

166. Maschino SE, Parnis SM, Buras WR, Guzman AW, inventors; Google Patents, assignee. Stimulating cranial nerve to treat disorders associated with the thyroid gland. 2010. https://www.google.com/patents/US7706874.

167. Parnis S, Maschino S, Buras W, Guzman A. Stimulating cranial nerve to treat pulmonary disorder. Google Patents; 2007. http://www.google.com.gt/patents/US20070027496.

168. Parnis SM, Maschino SE, Guzman AW. Cranial nerve stimulation to treat a vocal cord disorder. Google Patents; 2010. http://www.google.com/patents/US7840280.

169. Zabara J, Barrett BT, Parnis SM. Nerve stimulation as a treatment for pain. Google Patents; 2003. https://www.google.com/patents/WO2003063959A1?cl=en.

170. Phone interview with Madris Tomes, July 18, 2016.

171. Chudnoff SG, Nichols JE, Jr., Levie M. Hysteroscopic Essure inserts for permanent contraception: extended follow-up results of a phase III multicenter international study. *J Minim Invasive Gynecol.* 2015;22(6):951–960. http://www.ncbi.nlm.nih.gov/pubmed/25917278.

172. Casey J, Yunker A. Pelvic pain associated with Essure perforation. *J Minim Invasive Gynecol.* 2016;23(3):292.

173. Casey J, Aguirre F, Yunker A. Outcomes of laparoscopic removal of the Essure sterilization device for pelvic pain: a case series. *Contraception.* 2016;94(2):190–192.

174. Barbosa MW, Sotiriadis A, Papatheodorou SI, Mijatovic V, Nastri CO, Martins WP. High miscarriage rate in women submitted to Essure for hydrosalpinx before embryo transfer: a systematic review and meta-analysis. *Ultrasound Obstet Gynecol.* 2016;48(5):556–565.

175. Mao J, Pfeifer S, Schlegel P, Sedrakyan A. Safety and efficacy of hysteroscopic sterilization compared with laparoscopic sterilization: an observational cohort study. *BMJ.* 2015;351:h5162. http://www.ncbi.nlm.nih.gov/pubmed/26462857.

176. Food and Drug Administration Center for Devices and Radiological Health Obstetrics and Gynecology Devices Panel materials archive. 2002. http://www.accessdata.fda.gov/scripts/cdrh/cfdocs/cfadvisory/details.cfm?mtg=330.

177. Gariepy AM, Xu X, Creinin MD, Schwarz EB, Smith KJ. Hysteroscopic Essure inserts for permanent contraception: extended follow-up results of a phase III multicenter international study. *J Minim Invasive Gynecol.* 2016;23(1):137–138. https://www.ncbi.nlm.nih.gov/pubmed/26260301.

178. Awford J. "If 20,000 penises were falling off, the world would stop": Erin Brockovich backs women who claim a commercial contraceptive has left them in agony and needing abortions. *Daily Mail Australia* 2015. http://www.dailymail.co.uk/news/article-3298878/Erin-Brockovich-joins-campaign-pull-Essure-contraceptive-market.html#ixzz4K2Hsotaq.

179. Letter from Dayle Cristinzio, acting associate commissioner for legislation, FDA, to the Honorable Michael G. Fitzpatrick. 2016.

180. Letter from Jay Winckler, Winckler & Harvey, LLP, to Dennis Fegan, May 12, 2008.

181. *Riegel v. Medtronic* oral argument. Cornell University Law School Legal Information Institute. Dec 4, 2007. https://www.law.cornell.edu/supct/cert/06-179.

182. *Riegel v. Medtronic* US Supreme Court ruling. Feb 20, 2008. https://www.supremecourt.gov/opinions/07pdf/06-179.pdf.

183. Mencimer S. Daniel Troy's poison pill. *Mother Jones* 2008. http://www.motherjones.com/politics/2008/03/daniel-troys-poison-pill.

184. DeVaney DB, Hamilton PA. The 10,000 pound gorilla: federal preemption in class III medical device cases. *Florida Bar Journal* 2006. http://www.thefreelibrary.com/The+10%2c000+pound+gorilla%3a+federal+preemption+in+class+III+medical...-a0152762815.

185. McGarity TO. The perils of preemption. *Trial* 2008.

186. FDA history part iv: regulating cosmetics, devices, and veterinary medicine after 1938. http://www.fda.gov/AboutFDA/WhatWeDo/History/Origin/ucm055137.htm.

187. Sivin I. Another look at the Dalkon Shield: meta-analysis underscores its problems. *Contraception*. 1993;48(1):1–12.

188. Cox ML. The Dalkon Shield saga. *J Fam Plann Reprod Health Care*. 2003;29(1):8. https://www.ncbi.nlm.nih.gov/pubmed/12626170.

189. Daniel Schultz resigns amid CDRH controversies. *MDDI News* 2009. http://www.mddionline.com/article/daniel-schultz-resigns-amid-cdrh-controversies.

190. Garber AM. Modernizing device regulation. *N Engl J Med*. 2010;362(13):1161–1163. http://content.nejm.org/cgi/reprint/362/13/1161.pdf.

191. Zuckerman D, Brown P, Das A. Lack of publicly available scientific evidence on the safety and effectiveness of implanted medical devices. *JAMA Intern Med*. 2014;174(11):1781–1787. http://dx.doi.org/10.1001/jamainternmed.2014.4193.

192. *Medtronic, Inc. v. Lohr.* Cornell University Law School Legal Information Institute. 1996. https://www.law.cornell.edu/supct/html/95-754.ZS.html.

193. Phone interview with Vinay Prasad, August 1, 2016.

194. US Food and Drug Administration. List of device recalls. http://www.fda.gov/MedicalDevices/Safety/ListofRecalls/default.htm.

195. US Food and Drug Administration. PMA supplements and amendments. http://www.fda.gov/MedicalDevices/DeviceRegulationandGuidance/HowtoMarketYourDevice/PremarketSubmissions/PremarketApprovalPMA/ucm050467.htm.

196. Sperling MR. Sudden unexplained death in epilepsy. *Epilepsy Currents*. 2001;1(1):21–23. http://www.ncbi.nlm.nih.gov/pmc/articles/PMC320690/.

197. Gordon A. The Delicate Dance of Immersion and Insulation: The Politicization of the FDA Commissioner. 2003. https://dash.harvard.edu/bitstream/handle/1/8852141/Gordon.html?sequence=2.

198. Phone interview with Larry Kessler, October 24, 2016.

199. Silverman E. The FDA "revolving door" fosters conflicts on advisory panels. *Wall Street Journal Blog* 2014. http://blogs.wsj.com/pharmalot/2014/09/15/the-fda-revolving-door-fosters-conflicts-on-advisory-panels/.

200. Escobar C. He's back! Former VP at Monsanto to advise FDA commissioner on food safety. *Huffington Post* 2011. http://www.huffingtonpost.com/christine-escobar/hes-back-former-vp-at-mon_b_228792.html.

201. Carome M. Outrage of the month: revolving door at FDA undermines public confidence. Public Citizen. 2014. http://www.citizen.org/Page.aspx?pid=6298.

202. Lenzer J. Robert Califf: controversial new head of the FDA. *BMJ*. July 5, 2016 10:36:07, 2016;354. http://www.bmj.com/content/354/bmj.i3656.

203. Lenzer J. Bush plans to screen whole US population for mental illness. *BMJ*. 2004;328(7454):1458. http://www.bmj.com/content/328/7454/1458.1.

204. McGarity TO. *Bending Science: How Special Interests Corrupt Public Health Research*. Cambridge, MA: Harvard University Press; 2008.

205. Scott BG, Strickland EK. Recent developments in federal preemption of pharmaceutical drug and medical device product liability claims. *The Defender* 2009. http://www.spilmanlaw.com/media%20content/media-content/documents/preemption-developments.pdf.

206. Lenzer J. Doctors join protest over change to FDA rules on conflict of interest. *BMJ*. 2011;343:d5269. http://www.ncbi.nlm.nih.gov/pubmed/21852346.

207. Lenzer J. FDA is criticised for hinting it may loosen conflict of interest rules. *BMJ*. 2011;343:d5070. http://www.ncbi.nlm.nih.gov/pubmed/21824909.

208. Lenzer J. FDA bars own expert from evaluating risks of painkillers. *BMJ*. 2004;329(7476):1203. http://bmj.bmjjournals.com/cgi/content/full/329/7476/1203?ehom.

209. Harris G. New study links Pfizer's Bextra, similar to Vioxx, to heart attacks. *New York Times* 2004. http://www.nytimes.com/2004/11/10/business/new-study-links-pfizers-bextra-similar-to-vioxx-to-heart-attacks.html?_r=0.

210. Lenzer J. When is a point of view a conflict of interest? *BMJ*. 2016;355. http://www.bmj.com/content/bmj/355/bmj.i6194.full.pdf.

211. Steinbrook R. Financial conflicts of interest and the Food and Drug Administration's advisory committees. *N Engl J Med*. 2005;353(2):116–118. http://www.nejm.org/doi/full/10.1056/NEJMp058108.

212. Lurie P. Financial conflicts of interest are related to voting patterns at FDA advisory committee meetings. *MedGenMed*. 2006;8(4):22–22. http://www.ncbi.nlm.nih.gov/pmc/articles/PMC1868362/.

213. Lenzer J, Epstein K. The Yaz men: members of FDA panel reviewing the risks of popular Bayer contraceptive had industry ties. *Washington Monthly* 2012. http://www.washingtonmonthly.com/ten-miles-square/2012/01/the_yaz_men_members_of_fda_pan034651.php.

214. 2012 presidential race: health sector totals to candidates. Center for Responsive Politics. http://www.opensecrets.org/pres12/sectors.php?sector=H.

215. Greenfieldboyce N. FDA to fund controversial research foundation. *All Things Considered* 2012. http://www.npr.org/sections/health-shots/2012/04/03/149931282/fda-to-fund-controversial-research-foundation.

216. Johnson JA. The FDA Medical Device User Fee Program: MDUFA IV Reauthorization. 2016. https://www.fas.org/sgp/crs/misc/R44517.pdf.

217. Partnership for Public Service. The State of the FDA Workforce. 2012. https://ourpublicservice.org/publications/viewcontentdetails.php?id=43.

218. Mandrola J. Double counting…*DrJohnM*. http://www.drjohnm.org/2010/07/double-counting/.

219. Groeger L. Four medical implants that escaped FDA scrutiny. *ProPublica* 2012. https://www.propublica.org/special/four-medical-implants-that-escaped-fda-scrutiny.

220. Layton L. FDA look again at knee implant after reports of pressure. *Washington Post* 2009.

http://www.washingtonpost.com/wp-dyn/content/article/2009/09/24/
AR2009092404272.html.

221. Harris G, Halbfinger DM. F.D.A. reveals it fell to a push by lawmakers. *New York Times*
2009. http://www.nytimes.com/2009/09/25/health/policy/25knee.html?_r=0.

222. Ivy Sports Medicine has first implantation of the collagen meniscus implant (CMI). 2015.
http://www.ivysportsmed.com/en/about-us/news.

223. University of Michigan Fast Forward Medical Innovation. FDA Regulation of Medical Devices (Part 1 of 3). 2015. https://www.youtube.com/watch?v=yZAG5logVhE.

224. Institute of Medicine. *Medical Devices and the Public's Health: The FDA 510(k) Clearance Process at 35 Years.* Washington, DC: National Academies Press; 2011.

225. Letter to President Obama from FDA physicians, scientists. 2009. https://www.finance.
senate.gov/ranking-members-news/letter-to-president-obama-from-fda-physicians-scientists.

226. *Hardy v. Shuren*: second amended complaint. Case number 1:11-CV-01739-RLW. United States
District Court for the District of Columbia; 2012. legaltimes.typepad.com/files/fda2.pdf.

227. Zuckerman D. Why the 21st Century Cures Act could be disastrous for medicine.
National Center for Health Research. 2016. http://www.center4research.org/21st-century-
cures-act-disastrous-medicine/.

228. Lenzer J. Manufacturers tell FDA why they should be able to promote drugs and devices
off label. *BMJ.* 2016;355. http://www.bmj.com/content/bmj/355/bmj.i6098.full.pdf.

229. Spencer J, Carlson J. In letter to Franken, FDA defends handling of Medtronic's Infuse
study. *StarTribune* 2016. http://www.startribune.com/in-letter-to-franken-fda-defends-
handling-of-medtronic-s-infuse-study/384052101/.

230. Lenzer J. Watching over the medical device industry. *BMJ.* 2009;338:b2321. http://
www.bmj.com/cgi/content/full/338/jun23_1/b2321?view=long&pmid=19549649.

231. Lenzer J. Is the United States Preventive Services Task Force still a voice of caution? *BMJ.*
2017;356. http://www.bmj.com/content/bmj/356/bmj.j743.full.pdf.

232. Novella S. The role of anecdotes in science-based medicine. *Science-Based Medicine* 2008.
https://sciencebasedmedicine.org/the-role-of-anecdotes-in-science-based-medicine/.

233. Kosko J, Klassen TP, Bishop T, Hartling L. Evidence-based medicine and the anecdote:
uneasy bedfellows or ideal couple? *Paediatr Child Health.* 2006;11(10):665–668.
http://www.ncbi.nlm.nih.gov/pmc/articles/PMC2528597/.

234. Shukla GP, Asuri N. Natural history of temporal lobe epilepsy: antecedents and progression. *Epilepsy Research and Treatment.* 2012;2012. http://dx.doi.org/10.1155/2012/195073.

235. Kwan P, Sander JW. The natural history of epilepsy: an epidemiological view. *J Neurol, Neuro-
surg Psychiatry.* 2004;75(10):1376–1381. http://jnnp.bmj.com/content/75/10/1376.abstract.

236. Barrette S, Bernstein ML, Leclerc JM, et al. Treatment complications in children diagnosed with neuroblastoma during a screening program. *J Clin Oncol.*
2006;24(10):1542–1545. http://jco.ascopubs.org/cgi/content/abstract/24/10/1542.

237. Tsubono Y, Hisamichi S. A halt to neuroblastoma screening in Japan. *N Engl J Med.*
2004;350(19):2010–2011. http://www.nejm.org/doi/full/10.1056/NEJM200405063501922.

238. Woods WG, Gao RN, Shuster JJ, et al. Screening of infants and mortality due to neuroblastoma. *N Engl J Med.* 2002;346(14):1041–1046. http://content.nejm.org/cgi/content/
abstract/346/14/1041.

239. Prasad V, Rho J, Cifu A. The inferior vena cava filter: how could a medical device be
so well accepted without any evidence of efficacy? *JAMA Intern Med.* 2013;173(7):493–495.
http://dx.doi.org/10.1001/jamainternmed.2013.2725.

240. Terra VC, Furlanetti LL, Nunes AA, et al. Vagus nerve stimulation in pediatric patients: is it really worthwhile? *Epilepsy Behav.* 2014;31:329–333. http://www.ncbi.nlm.nih.gov/pubmed/24210463.

241. Cyberonics Physician's Manual VNS Therapy. 1997:240.

242. Gigerenzer G, Gaissmaier W, Kurz-Milcke E, Schwartz LM, Woloshin S. Helping doctors and patients make sense of health statistics. *Psychol Sci.* 2007;8(2):53–96. http://library.mpib-berlin.mpg.de/ft/gg/GG_Helping_2008.pdf.

243. Transmyocardial laser revascularization. *N Engl J Med.* 2000;342(6):436–438. http://www.nejm.org/doi/full/10.1056/NEJM200002103420615.

244. Briones E, Lacalle JR, Marin-Leon I, Rueda J-R. Transmyocardial laser revascularization versus medical therapy for refractory angina. *Cochrane Database Syst Rev.* 2015(2). http://dx.doi.org/10.1002/14651858.CD003712.pub3.

245. Musial F, Klosterhalfen S, Enck P. Placebo responses in patients with gastrointestinal disorders. *World J Gastroenterol.* 2007;13(25):3425–3429. http://www.ncbi.nlm.nih.gov/pmc/articles/PMC4146777/.

246. Jacoby VL, Subak L, Waetjen L. The FDA and the vaginal mesh controversy—further impetus to change the 510(k) pathway for medical device approval. *JAMA Intern Med.* 2016;176(2):277–278. http://dx.doi.org/10.1001/jamainternmed.2015.7155.

247. Cyberonics. Brief Summary of Safety Information for the VNS Therapy System [Epilepsy and Depression Indications] (March 2007). http://dynamic.cyberonics.com/manuals/doc_download.asp?docid=1380E48A-8094-4D9F-AA9A-22E5466435D1.

248. Cyberonics. Physician's Manual VNS Therapy Pulse Model 102 Generator and VNS Therapy Pulse Duo Model 102R Generator. 2003. https://www.fda.gov/ohrms/dockets/ac/04/briefing/4047b1_03_Epilepsy%20Physician%27s%20Manual.pdf.

249. Glorioso C, Schlesinger J, Stulberger E. Health companies label thousands of patient deaths as "injuries." CNBC. 2016. http://www.cnbc.com/2016/08/19/health-companies-label-thousands-of-patient-deaths-as-injuries.html.

250. Lenzer J. FOIA Request: FDA response to inquiry by Senator Solomon P. Ortiz re: VNS investigation; post-surveillance studies Jan 1, 1997 through May 16, 2016.

251. E-mails from Celeste Smith, Deputy Agency Chief, FOIA Officer, Aug 16, 17, and 23, 2016.

252. Labar D. Vagus nerve stimulation for 1 year in 269 patients on unchanged antiepileptic drugs. *Seizure.* 2004;13(6):392–398. PM:15276142.

253. Renfroe JB, Wheless JW. Earlier use of adjunctive vagus nerve stimulation therapy for refractory epilepsy. *Neurology.* 2002;59(90064):26S–30. http://www.neurology.org/cgi/content/abstract/59/6_suppl_4/S26.

254. Labar DR. Antiepileptic drug use during the first 12 months of vagus nerve stimulation therapy: a registry study. *Neurology.* 2002;59(90064):38S–43. http://www.neurology.org/cgi/content/abstract/59/6_suppl_4/S38.

255. Helmers SL, Griesemer DA, Dean JC, et al. Observations on the use of vagus nerve stimulation earlier in the course of pharmacoresistant epilepsy: patients with seizures for six years or less. *Neurologist.* 2003;9(3):160–164.

256. Amar AP, Apuzzo MLJ, Liu CY. Vagus nerve stimulation therapy after failed cranial surgery for intractable epilepsy: results from the vagus nerve stimulation therapy patient outcome registry. *Neurosurgery.* 2004;55(5). http://journals.lww.com/neurosurgery/Fulltext/2004/11000/Vagus_Nerve_Stimulation_Therapy_after_Failed.10.aspx.

257. Annegers JF, Coan SP, Hauser WA, Leestma J. Epilepsy, vagal nerve stimulation by the NCP system, all-cause mortality, and sudden, unexpected, unexplained death. *Epilepsia.* 2000;41(5):549–553. http://onlinelibrary.wiley.com/doi/10.1111/j.1528-1157.2000.tb00208.x/pdf

258. Scherrmann J, Hoppe C, Kral T, Schramm J, Elger CE. Vagus nerve stimulation: clinical experience in a large patient series. *J Clin Neurophysiol.* 2001;18(5):408–414.

259. Hoppe C. Vagus nerve stimulation: urgent need for the critical reappraisal of clinical effectiveness. *Seizure.* 2013;22(1):83–84. http://dx.doi.org/10.1016/j.seizure.2012.10.001.

260. Hoppe C, Helmstaedter C, Elger CE. Vagus nerve stimulation for epilepsy treatment in children. *Epilepsia.* 2015;56(2):323–324. https://www.ncbi.nlm.nih.gov/pubmed/25708479.

261. Hoppe C, Wagner L, Hoffman J, von Lehe M, Elger CE. Comprehensive long-term outcome of best drug treatment with or without add-on vagus nerve stimulation for epilepsy: a retrospective matched pairs case-control study. *Seizure.* 2013;22:109–115. https://pdfs.semanticscholar.org/e39d/1e9500ef7110a7e9f4d8a416172096c9cb92.pdf.

262. Bernstein AL, Barkan H, Hess T. Vagus nerve stimulation therapy for pharmacoresistant epilepsy: effect on health care utilization. *Epilepsy Behav.* 2007;10(1):134–137. http://www.epilepsybehavior.com/article/S1525-5050(06)00400-8/pdf.

263. Learmonth ID, Young C, Rorabeck C. The operation of the century: total hip replacement. *Lancet.* 2007;370(9597):1508–1519.

264. Tower S. Hip metallosis and corrosion—a million harmed due to FDA inaction. *J Patient Saf.* Nov 02, 2016. https://www.ncbi.nlm.nih.gov/pubmed/27811592.

265. Tower SS. Arthroprosthetic cobaltism associated with metal on metal hip implants. *BMJ.* Jan 17, 2012;344:e430. https://www.ncbi.nlm.nih.gov/pubmed/22252702.

266. Machado C, Appelbe A, Wood R. Arthroprosthetic cobaltism and cardiomyopathy. *Heart Lung Circ.* 2012;21(11):759–60. https://www.ncbi.nlm.nih.gov/pubmed/22520206.

267. Roessler PP, Witt F, Efe T, Schmitt J. Arthroprosthetic cobaltism and pseudotumour also occur in patients with small diameter femoral ball head metal-on-metal total hip arthroplasties. *BMJ Case Rep.* Mar 28, 2014;2014. https://www.ncbi.nlm.nih.gov/pubmed/24682139.

268. Gessner BD, Steck T, Woelber E, Tower SS. A systematic review of systemic cobaltism after wear or corrosion of chrome-cobalt hip implants. *J Patient Saf.* Jun 12, 2015. https://www.ncbi.nlm.nih.gov/pubmed/26076080.

269. Tower SS. Cobalt toxicity in two hip replacement patients. *State of Alaska Epidemiology Bulletin.* 2010. www.epi.alaska.gov/bulletins/docs/b2010_14.pdf.

270. DePuy ASR recall issued after warning about hip replacement failures. 2010. http://www.aboutlawsuits.com/depuy-asr-recall-hip-replacement-failures-12276/.

271. Feeley J. J&J to pay as much as $420 million more in ASR hip accord. *Bloomberg News* 2015. http://www.bloomberg.com/news/articles/2015-02-23/j-j-to-pay-as-much-as-420-million-more-in-asr-hip-accord.

272. Michel R, Nolte M, Reich M, Loer F. Systemic effects of implanted prostheses made of cobalt-chromium alloys. *Arch Orthop Trauma Surg.* 1991;110(2):61–74.

273. Sunderman FW, Jr., Hopfer SM, Swift T, et al. Cobalt, chromium, and nickel concentrations in body fluids of patients with porous-coated knee or hip prostheses. *J Orthop Res.* 1989;7(3):307–315.

274. International Medical Device Regulators Forum. Patient Registry: Essential Principles. 2015. http://www.imdrf.org/docs/imdrf/final/consultations/imdrf-cons-essential-principles-151124.pdf.

275. European Commission. Final opinion on metal-on-metal joint replacements. 2014. https://ec.europa.eu/health/scientific_committees/consultations/public_consultations/scenihr_consultation_20_en.

276. Allen LA, Ambardekar AV, Devaraj KM, Maleszewski JJ, Wolfel EE. Missing elements of the history. *N Engl J Med.* 2014;370(6):559–566. http://www.nejm.org/doi/full/10.1056/NEJMcps1213196.

277. Wise J. TV show *House* helped doctors spot cobalt poisoning. *BMJ.* 2014;348. http://www.bmj.com/content/bmj/348/bmj.g1424.full.pdf.

278. Dahms K, Sharkova Y, Heitland P, Pankuweit S, Schaefer JR. Cobalt intoxication diagnosed with the help of Dr House. *Lancet.* 2014;383(9916):574. https://www.ncbi.nlm.nih.gov/pubmed/24506908.

279. E-mail from William Maisel to Stephen Tower. April 30, 2012.

280. Meier B. Johnson & Johnson in Deal to Settle Hip Implant Lawsuits. *New York Times* 2013. http://www.nytimes.com/2013/11/20/business/johnson-johnson-to-offer-2-5-billion-hip-device-settlement.html

281. Pijls BG, Meessen JMTA, Schoones JW, et al. Increased mortality in metal-on-metal versus non-metal-on-metal primary total hip arthroplasty at 10 years and longer follow-up: a systematic review and meta-analysis. *PLoS One.* 2016;11(6):e0156051. http://dx.doi.org/10.1371%2Fjournal.pone.0156051.

282. Phone interviews with Dr. Kathleen Yaremchuk, May 25, 2016, and February 25, 2017.

283. Yaremchuk KL, Toma MS, Somers ML, Peterson E. Acute airway obstruction in cervical spinal procedures with bone morphogenetic proteins. *Laryngoscope.* 2010;120(10):1954–1957. https://www.ncbi.nlm.nih.gov/pubmed/20824786.

284. MAUDE report "Infuse" death. 12/12/2008. http://www.accessdata.fda.gov/scripts/cdrh/cfdocs/cfMAUDE/detail.cfm?mdrfoi__id=1289583.

285. Buchowski JM, Riew KD, Nussenbaum B. In reference to "Acute airway obstruction in cervical spinal procedures with bone morphogenetic proteins." *Laryngoscope.* 2011;121(11):2501; author reply 2502–2503. https://www.ncbi.nlm.nih.gov/pubmed/21898420.

286. Greene J. Doctor creates system to put limits on sales representatives. *Crain's Detroit Business* 2009. http://www.crainsdetroit.com/print/article/20090809/AWARDS05/308099992/doctor-creates-system-to-put-limits-on-sales-representatives.

287. Epstein NE, Schwall GS. Costs and frequency of "off-label" use of INFUSE for spinal fusions at one institution in 2010. *Surg Neurol Int.* 2011;2:115. https://www.ncbi.nlm.nih.gov/pubmed/21886888.

288. FDA public health notification: life-threatening complications associated with recombinant human bone morphogenetic protein in cervical spine fusion. 2008. http://www.fda.gov/MedicalDevices/Safety/AlertsandNotices/PublicHealthNotifications/ucm062000.htm.

289. Epstein NE. Complications due to the use of BMP/INFUSE in spine surgery: the evidence continues to mount. *Surg Neurol Int.* 2013;4(Suppl 5):S343–352. https://www.ncbi.nlm.nih.gov/pubmed/23878769.

290. Carragee EJ, Hurwitz EL, Weiner BK. A critical review of recombinant human bone morphogenetic protein-2 trials in spinal surgery: emerging safety concerns and lessons learned. *Spine J.* 2011;11(6):471–491. http://dx.doi.org/10.1016/j.spinee.2011.04.023.

291. Carragee EJ, Chu G, Rohatgi R, et al. Cancer risk after use of recombinant bone mor-

phogenetic protein-2 for spinal arthrodesis. *J Bone Joint Surg Am.* 2013;95(17):1537–1545. http://jbjs.org/content/jbjsam/95/17/1537.full.pdf.

292. Devine JG, Dettori JR, France JC, Brodt E, McGuire RA. The use of rhBMP in spine surgery: is there a cancer risk? *Evid Based Spine Care J.* May, 2012;3(2):35–41. https://www.ncbi.nlm.nih.gov/pubmed/23230416.

293. *Lew v. Medtronic.* Case number CV 14-08303-JLS (VBKx). United States District Court for the Central District of California; 2014. http://www.leagle.com/decision/In%20FDCO%2020141217940/Lew%20v.%20Medtronic,%20Inc

295. Rubenstein S. Grassley points to another academic doctor's industry pay. *Wall Street Journal Health Blog* 2009. http://blogs.wsj.com/health/2009/05/28/grassley-points-to-another-academic-doctors-pay-from-industry/.

296. Terhune C. UC OKs paying surgeon $10 million in whistleblower-retaliation case. *Los Angeles Times* 2014. http://www.latimes.com/business/la-fi-ucla-doctor-conflicts-20140423-story.html.

297. Terhune C. Regents OK $8.5 million for 2 patients suing over financial conflicts at UCLA. *Los Angeles Times* 2016. http://www.latimes.com/business/la-fi-ucla-wang-medtronics-20160729-snap-story.html.

298. *Jerome Lew v. Jeffrey C. Wang, M.D.* Regents of the University of California case number: SC120518, Superior Court of the State of California, County of Los Angeles, Central District.

299. Phone interview with Nancy Epstein, May 24, 2016.

300. Epstein NE. Are recommended spine operations either unnecessary or too complex? Evidence from second opinions. *Surg Neurol Int.* 2013;4(Suppl 5):S353–358. https://www.ncbi.nlm.nih.gov/pubmed/24340231.

301. Phone interview with Eugene J. Carragee, May 5, 2016.

302. Fauber J. Senators investigate Medtronic spine device. *Milwaukee Journal Sentinel* 2011. http://www.medpagetoday.com/surgery/orthopedics/27200.

303. Staff report on Medtronic's influence on INFUSE clinical studies. *Int J Occup Environ Health.* 2013;19(2):67–76. http://dx.doi.org/10.1179/2049396713Y.0000000020.

304. Moore J. Suit alleges that Medtronic tried to entice doctors to use its device. *StarTribune.* Dec 11, 2008.

305. Young R. Carragee must resign. *Orthopedics This Week* 2013. https://ryortho.com/2013/06/dr-eugene-carragee-must-resign/.

306. Spencer J, Carlson J, Webster M. Question of risk: Medtronic's lost study. *StarTribune* 2016. http://www.startribune.com/question-of-risk-medtronic's-lost-Infuse-study/372957441/.

307. Hustedt JW, Blizzard DJ. The controversy surrounding bone morphogenetic proteins in the spine: a review of current research. *Yale J Biol Med.* 2014;87(4):549–561. http://www.ncbi.nlm.nih.gov/pmc/articles/PMC4257039/.

308. *Andrew Hagerty v. Cyberonics, Inc.,* Aug 8, 2012 (United States District Court for the District of Massachusetts Case 1:12-cv-11465-FDS).

309. *United States of America et al. ex rel. Andrew Hagerty v. Cyberonics, Inc.,* Civil No 13-10214-FDS, 3/31/2015 (United States District Court for the District of Massachusetts).

310. Carlat D. Dr. drug rep. *New York Times* 2007. http://www.nytimes.com/2007/11/25/magazine/25memoir-t.html?sq=daniel%20carlat%20shame&st=cse&scp=1&pagewanted=print.

311. Lenzer J, Brownlee S. Doctor takes "march of shame" to atone for drug company payments. *BMJ.* 2008;336(7634):20–21. http://www.bmj.com/cgi/content/full/336/7634/20.

312. Brownlee S, Lenzer J. Medical devices that can kill. *Reader's Digest* 2010. http://www.center4research.org/medical-devices-can-kill/.

313. Lenzer J, Brownlee S. An untold story? *BMJ*. 2008;336(7643):532–534. http://www.bmj.com/cgi/content/full/336/7643/532.

314. E-mail from William Maisel, MD, MPH, to Dennis Fegan, Dec 31, 2010.

315. Husten L. Cardiologist William Maisel arrested in prostitution sting operation. *Forbes* 2012. http://www.forbes.com/sites/larryhusten/2012/08/01/cardiologist-william-maisel-arrested-in-prostitution-sting-operation/#19a121eb397f.

316. Coronado O. Police incident report, Corpus Christi PD, dated 8/25/2013, regarding Dennis Fegan.

317. Letter from Jay L. Winckler, Winckler & Harvey, to Dennis Fegan, 2008.

319. Ehrhardt S, Appel LJ, Meinert CL. Trends in National Institutes of Health funding for clinical trials registered in clinicaltrials.gov. *JAMA*. 2015;314(23):2566–2567. http://dx.doi.org/10.1001/jama.2015.12206.

320. Krimsky S. *Science in the Private Interest: Has the Lure of Profits Corrupted Biomedical Research?* Lanham, MD: Rowman & Littlefield; 2004.

321. Benotti JR, Grossman W, Braunwald E, Davolos DD, Alousi AA. Hemodynamic assessment of amrinone. A new inotropic agent. *N Engl J Med*. 1978;299(25):1373–1377. https://www.ncbi.nlm.nih.gov/pubmed/714115.

322. Robbins RA. Profiles in medical courage: Peter Wilmshurst, the physician fugitive. *Southwest J Pulm Crit Care* 2012;4:134–141. http://www.swjpcc.com/general-medicine/2012/4/27/profiles-in-medical-courage-peter-wilmshurst-the-physician-f.html.

323. Smith R. A successful and cheerful whistleblower. *BMJ Blog* 2010. http://blogs.bmj.com/bmj/2012/10/10/richard-smith-a-successful-and-cheerful-whistleblower/.

324. Personal communication with Peter Wilmshurst.

325. Wilmshurst PT, Thompson DS, Juul SM, et al. Effects of intracoronary and intravenous amrinone infusions in patients with cardiac failure and patients with near normal cardiac function. *Br Heart J*. 1985;53(5):493–506. https://www.ncbi.nlm.nih.gov/pubmed/3994862.

326. Wilmshurst P. The politics of disclosure [letter; comment]. *Lancet*. 1997;349(9050):510. PM:0009040612.

327. Wilmshurst P. Obstacles to honesty in medical research. HealthWatch. 2003. https://www.healthwatch-uk.org/20-awards/award-lectures/65-2003-dr-peter-wilmshurst.html.

328. Massie B, Bourassa M, DiBianco R, et al. Long-term oral administration of amrinone for congestive heart failure: lack of efficacy in a multicenter controlled trial. *Circulation*. 1985;71(5):963–971. https://www.ncbi.nlm.nih.gov/pubmed/3886191.

329. Rettig G, Sen S, Frohlig G, Schieffer H, Bette L. Withdrawal of long-term amrinone therapy in patients with congestive heart failure: a placebo controlled trial. *Eur Heart J*. 1986;7(7):628–631. https://academic.oup.com/eurheartj/article-abstract/7/7/628/609047/Withdrawal-of-long-term-amrinone-therapy-in?redirectedFrom=PDF.

330. Erlichman J. Drug firm "made threats." Company tested heart drug with DHSS clearance. *The Guardian* 1986.

331. Boseley S. Warning signs on doctors' roadshow. *The Guardian* 2001. https://www.theguardian.com/society/2001/feb/15/uknews2.

332. Broad WJ. Notorious Darsee case shakes assumptions about science. *New York Times* 1983. https://scholar.google.com/scholar?cluster=13739026994092975982&hl=en&as_sdt=0,33.

333. Oransky O. Coming clean: a major figure in cardiology publishes a lengthy conflict of interest correction in JAMA. *Retraction Watch* 2012. http://retractionwatch.com/2012/02/

07/coming-clean-a-major-figure-in-cardiology-publishes-a-lengthy-conflict-of-interest-correction-in-jama/.

334. Wallis C. Fraud in a Harvard lab. *Time* 1983. http://content.time.com/time/magazine/article/0,9171,955142-1,00.html.

335. Dingell JD. Misconduct in medical research. *N Engl J Med*. 1993;328(22):1610–1615. http://www.nejm.org/doi/full/10.1056/NEJM199306033282207.

336. Boffey P. Study accusing researchers of inaccuracies is published. *New York Times* 1987. http://www.nytimes.com/1987/01/15/us/study-accusing-researchers-of-inaccuracies-is-published.html.

337. Boffey P. Major study points to faulty research at two universities. *New York Times* 1986. http://www.nytimes.com/1986/04/22/science/major-study-points-to-faulty-research-at-two-universities.html?pagewanted=all.

338. Stewart WW, Feder N. The integrity of the scientific literature. *Nature*. 1987;325(6101):207–214. https://www.ncbi.nlm.nih.gov/pubmed/3808019.

339. Braunwald E. On analyzing scientific fraud. *Nature*. 1987;325(6101):215–216.

340. Braunwald E, Kloner RA. Retraction of "Early recovery of regional performance in salvaged ischemic myocardium following coronary artery occlusion in the dog." *J Clin Invest*. 1982;70(4):following 915. https://www.ncbi.nlm.nih.gov/pubmed/6765636.

341. Bylinsky G. Genentech has a golden goose. *Fortune* 1988. http://archive.fortune.com/magazines/fortune/fortune_archive/1988/05/09/70518/index.htm.

342. Marsa L. *Prescription for Profits: How the Pharmaceutical Industry Bankrolled the Unholy Alliance Between Science and Business*. New York: Scribner; 1997.

343. E-mail from Genentech, August 25, 2016.

344. Stampfer MJ, Goldhaber SZ, Yusuf S, Peto R, Hennekens CH. Effect of intravenous streptokinase on acute myocardial infarction. *N Engl J Med*. 1982;307(19):1180–1182. http://www.nejm.org/doi/full/10.1056/NEJM198211043071904.

345. International Study Group. In-hospital mortality and clinical course of 20,891 patients with suspected acute myocardial infarction randomised between alteplase and streptokinase with or without heparin. *Lancet*. July 14, 1990, 1990;336(8707):71–75. http://www.sciencedirect.com/science/article/pii/0140673690915907.

346. Topol EJ, Morris DC, Smalling RW, et al. A multicenter, randomized, placebo-controlled trial of a new form of intravenous recombinant tissue-type plasminogen activator (activase) in acute myocardial infarction. *J Am Coll Cardiol*. 1987;9(6):1205–1213. http://www.sciencedirect.com/science/article/pii/S0735109787804576.

347. TIMI Study Group. The thrombolysis in myocardial infarction (TIMI) trial. *N Engl J Med*. 1985;312(14):932–936. http://www.nejm.org/doi/full/10.1056/NEJM198504043121437.

348. Bassler D, Briel M, Montori VM, et al. Stopping randomized trials early for benefit and estimation of treatment effects: systematic review and meta-regression analysis. *JAMA*. 2010;303(12):1180–1187. http://www.ncbi.nlm.nih.gov/pubmed/20332404.

349. Dalen JE, Gore JM, Braunwald E, et al. Six- and twelve-month follow-up of the phase I thrombolysis in myocardial infarction (TIMI) trial. *Am J Cardiol*. 1988;62(4):179–185. https://www.ncbi.nlm.nih.gov/pubmed/3135737.

350. Sherry S, Marder VJ. Creation of the recombinant tissue plasminogen activator (rt-PA) image and its influence on practice habits. *J Am Coll Cardiol*. 1991;18(6):1579–1582. https://www.ncbi.nlm.nih.gov/pubmed/1939964.

351. GISSI-2: a factorial randomised trial of alteplase versus streptokinase and heparin versus

no heparin among 12,490 patients with acute myocardial infarction. Gruppo Italiano per lo Studio della Sopravvivenza nell'Infarto Miocardico. *Lancet.* 1990;336(8707):65–71. https://www.ncbi.nlm.nih.gov/pubmed/1975321.

352. ISIS-3: a randomised comparison of streptokinase vs tissue plasminogen activator vs anistreplase and of aspirin plus heparin vs aspirin alone among 41,299 cases of suspected acute myocardial infarction. ISIS-3 (Third International Study of Infarct Survival) Collaborative Group. *Lancet.* 1992;339(8796):753–770. https://www.ncbi.nlm.nih.gov/pubmed/1347801.

353. Maatz CT. University physician-researcher conflicts of interest: the inadequacy of current controls and proposed reform. *Berkeley Technology Law Journal.* 1992;7(1). http://scholarship.law.berkeley.edu/cgi/viewcontent.cgi?article=1102&context=btlj.

354. O'Donnell M. Battle of the clotbusters. *BMJ.* 1991;302(6787):1259–1261. http://www.ncbi.nlm.nih.gov/pmc/articles/PMC1669945/.

355. Ridker PM, O'Donnell CJ, Marder VJ, Hennekens CH. A response to "holding gusto up to the light." *Ann Intern Med.* 1994;120(10):882–885. http://dx.doi.org/10.7326/0003-4819-120-10-199405150-00010.

356. Friedman HS. Streptokinase versus alteplase in acute myocardial infarction. *J R Soc Med.* 1996;89(8):427–430. https://www.ncbi.nlm.nih.gov/pubmed/8795494.

357. Blakeslee S. Health: cardiology; doctors split over best way to treat heart attack victims. *New York Times* 1989. http://www.nytimes.com/1989/03/23/us/health-cardiology-doctors-split-over-best-way-to-treat-heart-attack-victims.html?pagewanted=all&pagewanted=print.

358. Institute of Medicine. Clinical Trials in Cardiovascular Disease. In: Institute of Medicine. *Transforming Clinical Research in the United States: Challenges and Opportunities.* Washington, DC: National Academies Press; 2010.

359. Phone interview with Eugene Braunwald, January 28, 2013.

360. Wen P. Jurors outraged by psychiatrist's conduct. *Boston Globe* 2010. http://archive.boston.com/news/local/massachusetts/articles/2010/02/11/jurors_outraged_by_psychiatrists_conduct/.

361. Harris G, Carey B. Researchers fail to reveal full drug pay. *New York Times* 2008. http://www.nytimes.com/2008/06/08/us/08conflict.html.

362. Harris G. Top psychiatrist didn't report drug makers' pay. *New York Times* 2008. http://www.nytimes.com/2008/10/04/health/policy/04drug.html?_r=0.

363. Lenzer J. Review launched after Harvard psychiatrist failed to disclose industry funding. *BMJ.* 2008;336(7657):1327–1132a. http://www.bmj.com/cgi/content/short/336/7657/1327-a.

364. Podrid PJ, Graboys TB, Lown B. Prognosis of medically treated patients with coronary-artery disease with profound ST-segment depression during exercise testing. *N Engl J Med.* 1981;305(19):1111–1116. http://www.ncbi.nlm.nih.gov/pubmed/7290118.

365. Chan PS, Patel MR, Klein LW, et al. Appropriateness of percutaneous coronary intervention. *JAMA.* 2011;306(1):53–61. http://dx.doi.org/10.1001/jama.2011.916.

366. Gulba DC, Lichtlen PR. rt-PA versus streptokinase—has the controversy regarding the optimal thrombolytic agent been resolved by results of the GISSI II/International rt-PA vs. streptokinase fatality study? *Z Kardiol.* 1991;80(1):1–5. https://www.ncbi.nlm.nih.gov/pubmed/2035282.

367. Garattini S, Bertele V, Bertolini G. A failed attempt at collaboration. *BMJ.* 2013;347. http://www.bmj.com/content/bmj/347/bmj.f5354.full.pdf.

368. Lenzer J. Experts and activists discuss how to get "right care" for patients. *BMJ*. 2016-04-29 11:21:06, 2016;353. http://www.bmj.com/content/353/bmj.i2406.

369. Gawande A. The hot spotters: can we lower medical costs by giving the neediest patients better care? *New Yorker* 2011. http://www.newyorker.com/magazine/2011/01/24/the-hot-spotters.

370. Geyman J. Hijacked—stolen health care reform: why health care costs will not be contained. Physicians for a National Health Program. 2010. http://pnhp.org/blog/2010/07/08/hijacked-stolen-health-care-reform-why-health-care-costs-will-not-be-contained/.

371. Reid TR. *The Healing of America: A Global Quest for Better, Cheaper, and Fairer*. New York: Penguin Press; 2009.

372. Sinsky C, Colligan L, Li L, et al. Allocation of physician time in ambulatory practice: a time and motion study in 4 specialties. *Ann Intern Med*. 2016;165(11):753–760. http://dx.doi.org/10.7326/M16-0961.

373. Woolhandler S, Himmelstein DU. Administrative work consumes one-sixth of U.S. physicians' working hours and lowers their career satisfaction. *Int J Health Serv*. 2014;44(4):635–642. https://www.ncbi.nlm.nih.gov/pubmed/25626223.

374. Shapiro J. France's model health care for new mothers. *Morning Edition*. 2008. http://www.npr.org/templates/story/story.php?storyId=92116914.

375. Geyman J. The takeover of U. S. health care by big money. *Huffington Post Blog* 2017. http://www.huffingtonpost.com/john-geyman/the-takeover-of-u-s-healt_b_13939088.html.

376. Gaffney A, Woolhandler S, Angell M, Himmelstein DU. Moving forward from the Affordable Care Act to a single-payer system. *Am J Public Health*. 2016;106(6):987–988. https://www.ncbi.nlm.nih.gov/pubmed/27148891.

377. Potter W. Cry me a river, Aetna. Moyers & Company. 2016. http://billmoyers.com/story/cry-river-aetna/.

378. Lenzer J. Psychiatrists urge Obama to request neuropsychiatric review of Trump. *BMJ*. 2016;355. http://www.bmj.com/content/bmj/355/bmj.i6775.full.pdf.

379. DiJulio B, Firth J, Kirzinger A, Brodie M. Kaiser health tracking poll: February 2016. Henry J. Kaiser Family Foundation. http://kff.org/global-health-policy/poll-finding/kaiser-health-tracking-poll-february-2016/.

380. Ariely D, Gneezy U, Loewenstein G, Mazar N. Large stakes and big mistakes. *Review of Economic Studies*. 2009;76(2):451–469.

381. Project on Government Oversight. The FDA's Deadly Gamble with the Safety of Medical Devices. 2009. http://www.pogo.org/pogo-files/reports/public-health/safety-of-medical-devices/ph-fda-20090218.html

382. Mukherjee S. Trump is slashing FDA rules. Why isn't big pharma excited? *Fortune* 2017. http://fortune.com/2017/03/28/trump-fda-regulations-drug-policy/.

383. Lenzer J, Hoffman JR, Furberg CD, Ioannidis JP. Ensuring the integrity of clinical practice guidelines: a tool for protecting patients. *BMJ*. 2013;347:f5535. http://www.ncbi.nlm.nih.gov/pubmed/24046286.

384. Morris AH, Ioannidis JP. Limitations of medical research and evidence at the patient-clinician encounter scale. *Chest*. 2013;143(4):1127–1135. http://www.ncbi.nlm.nih.gov/pubmed/23546485.

385. Anderson JF. Secrecy in the courts: at the tipping point. *Villanova Law Review*. 2008;53(5). http://digitalcommons.law.villanova.edu/cgi/viewcontent.cgi?article=1123&context=vlr.

386. Rasor D. Confidentiality settlements hide dangerous corporate behavior. Truthout.

http://www.truth-out.org/article/item/471:confidentiality-settlements-hide-dangerous-corporate-behavior.

387. Board E. Secrecy that kills. *New York Times* 2014. https://www.nytimes.com/2014/06/01/opinion/sunday/secrecy-that-kills.html?_r=0.

388. Givelber DJ, Robbins A. Public health versus court sponsored secrecy. *Law & Contemporary Problems.* 2006;69:131–139. scholarship.law.duke.edu/cgi/viewcontent.cgi?article=1390&context=lcp.

389. Marmot MG, Stansfeld S, Patel C, et al. Health inequalities among British civil servants: the Whitehall II study. *Lancet.* 1991;337(8754):1387–1393. http://dx.doi.org/10.1016/0140-6736(91)93068-K.

390. Thompson D. Get rich, live longer: the ultimate consequence of income inequality. *The Atlantic* 2014. http://www.theatlantic.com/business/archive/2014/04/more-money-more-life-the-depressing-reality-of-inequality-in-america/360895/.

391. McKinlay JB, McKinlay SM. The questionable contribution of medical measures to the decline of mortality in the United States in the twentieth century. *Milbank Memorial Fund Quarterly. Health and Society.* 1977;55(3):405–428. http://www.columbia.edu/itc/hs/pubhealth/rosner/g8965/client_edit/readings/week_2/mckinlay.pdf.

392. Bezruchka S. Inequality kills. *Boston Review* 2014. http://www.bostonreview.net/us/stephen-bezruchka-inequality-kills.

393. Halfon N. The primacy of prevention. *The American Prospect* 2008. http://prospect.org/article/primacy-prevention.

394. Marmot M. Inequalities in health. *N Engl J Med.* 2001;345(2):134–136. http://www.nejm.org/doi/full/10.1056/NEJM200107123450210.

395. Shi C, Flanagan SR, Samadani U. Vagus nerve stimulation to augment recovery from severe traumatic brain injury impeding consciousness: a prospective pilot clinical trial. *Neurol Res.* 2013;35(3):263–276.

396. Tan A. Vagus Nerve Stimulation (VNS) and Rehabilitation in the Treatment of TBI. Fort Detrick, MD: U.S. Army Medical Research and Materiel Command; 2009. http://www.dtic.mil/dtic/tr/fulltext/u2/a504184.pdf.

Index

About the Author

Jeanne Lenzer is an award-winning medical investigative journalist and former Knight Science Journalism fellow. She is a longtime contributor to the *The BMJ* (formerly the *British Medical Journal*), and her articles, reviews, and commentary have appeared in the *New York Times Magazine*, *The Atlantic*, the *New Republic*, *Discover*, *Slate*, *Mother Jones*, and many other outlets.